Getting Through It

My Year of Cancer during Covid

Helen Epstein

Plunkett Lake Press

Plunkett Lake Press edition, 2022

ISBN 979-8-9851925-3-7

https://plunkettlakepress.com

Cover by Susan Erony

Praise for *Getting Through It*

"A memorable account of how a woman of parts received the dread diagnosis of cancer and taught herself to live with it. *Getting Through It* is both absorbing and admirable." – **Vivian Gornick, author of *The Situation and the Story* and *Unfinished Business***

"Helen Epstein's chronicle as told in *Getting Through It* is intimate and comprehensive. She reports and reflects on all aspects of cancer, from the factual to the existential. Cancer, like Covid, is both intensely communal and solitary. What a resource this book is – for cancer patients, yes, especially women. And for all of us who find ourselves living with and reflecting on, in Epstein's words, 'illness, death and new ways of coming back to life.'" – **Margo Jefferson, author of *Negroland* and *Constructing a Nervous System***

"A profoundly important book – not only for cancer patients, but for their families, friends, policy makers, and health care professionals. Epstein writes with breathtaking clarity about the challenges of undergoing treatment for a silent killer. Candid, compelling and psychologically astute." – **Helen Fremont, author of *After Long Silence* and *The Escape Artist***

"There are a lot of 'cancer memoirs' out there, but Helen Epstein has accomplished something singular – and far more useful. The candor is exemplary, the detail (including about the overwhelming confusion in the midst of the best care and research) is remarkable. This is the story of how not only a woman, but a marriage goes through a life-threatening ordeal. A must read not only for cancer patients and their caregivers, but for anyone (me, for example) who has frequent worried moments." – **Patricia Hampl, author of *The Art of the Wasted Day***

"In this eloquent narrative, journalist Helen Epstein brings her decades of skill to the tasks of chronicling the 'badge of illness' that a gynecological cancer diagnosis brought her. Unsparing in its measure of fear, chemically induced forgetting, and loss of control, we are treated to an honest appraisal of the cancer experience. This book is at once a reminder of our expectation of independence and the need for dependence that makes us deeply human." – **Susan M. Reverby, McLean Professor Emerita in the History of Ideas and Professor Emerita of Women's and Gender Studies, Wellesley College**

"Helen Epstein has a way of sharing intimate details of difficulties in her life that resonates with thousands of readers. Her no-holds-barred memoir and how-to of being diagnosed and treated for GYN cancer breaks many taboos in the medical and psychological conversation. Her page-turner of resilience will open up dialogue between patients, medical staff, friends and family members in this increasingly common part of 21st century life." – **Dr. Eva Fogelman, psychologist, author, and award-winning filmmaker of *Breaking the Silence: The Generation After the Holocaust***

"*Getting Through It* is my kind of self-help book, meaning it is not really a self-help book at all. In crystal clear prose, Epstein discusses her symptoms, her prognosis, her doctors, her nurses, her caregivers, her friendships, her diet, her sex life, her treatments and their side effects. Most astonishing is that despite its wrenching subject, *Getting Through It* is not a hard read. Epstein is so clear-eyed and sure-footed a narrator that the book manages to be comforting without being condescending, to be helpful without relying upon false hope." – **Laurel Leff, Professor, School of Journalism, Northeastern University, and author of *Well Worth Saving: American Universities Life-and-Death Decisions on Refugees from Nazi Europe***

"A fast read and eye-opening memoir that both doctors and patients will find valuable. Frank and funny, Epstein describes the myriad of life complexities, doubts, unanswered questions, and fears experienced by cancer patients and the people who love them." – **Audrey Konow, MD, Internist/Hospitalist, Providence St. Jude Medical Center**

"In this astonishingly candid book, Helen applies her laser focus to the day-to-day, sometimes minute-to-minute experience of cancer and its treatments during a pandemic. She describes a cast of fascinating doctors and nurses and the sometimes unexpected behavior of friends. Most beautiful is the inspiring portrait of her marriage with a partner who is there every step of the way. An enormously engaging, compulsively readable memoir." – **Susan Miron, Book Critic-at-Large**

"An unflinching, unsqueamish and eloquent account of cancer by a woman who beat it and can show the rest of us how it's done. Patients, friends and family of patients, and members of the medical profession will appreciate this acute, revealing report from the front lines." – **Dr. Cristina Nehring, author of *A Vindication of Love: Reclaiming Romance for the 21st Century***

"Over the course of a journalism career that has spanned five decades, Helen Epstein has explored what it means to be 'possessed by a past which one has not lived' as a child of Holocaust survivors. She has taken readers into the concert halls, dressing rooms and inner sanctums of some of our greatest artists and impresarios. Diagnosed with endometrial cancer in the early days of Covid pandemic lockdown, Helen turned her gimlet eye on herself as she, her loved ones and medical team moved through diagnosis, treatment and recovery. We journey with her through resurfaced memories and new routines, through unanticipated setbacks and unexpected pleasures. Through it all, we experience, again, what endures when all that we think we need to be who we are seems threatened. This book will stay with me for a long time." – **Kim Pearson, Associate Professor, Department of Journalism, The College of New Jersey**

Some women prefer to keep it private. Some want to know only what their doctors tell them. Others go online to learn everything they can. Many, like the women who got in touch with me after they heard I had endometrial cancer, want to hear how another woman got through treatment and came out standing. This book is for all of them.

April 2020

When the pandemic hit Boston, I canceled my routine medical check-ups – eye, dental, and an already twice-postponed pelvic ultrasound. Like so many other people, I weighed the risks of contracting Covid and decided against a routine medical visit. I'm a medical minimalist, the opposite of my husband, who calls his physician whenever he has a cold. The only doctor I consult without fail, whenever I have a hint of a problem, is my gynecologist.

Despite changes in health plans and a retirement, I have had consistently good gynecologists, who helped me through two miscarriages, delivered my two sons and kept an eye on my four persistent uterine fibroids. Dr. Martha Richardson was the last one I saw regularly. She was about my age, meticulous, collaborative, and took her time with patients. When we were in our mid-50s, and I complained of trouble sleeping, dry eyes, dry skin, dry everything genital, we discussed the many research studies on hormone replacement therapy. In my case, the pros outweighed the cons. She prescribed it, and added pelvic ultrasounds to my schedule of mammograms and Pap smears.

Every few years, she ordered a special, trans-vaginal pelvic ultrasound to monitor the thickness of my uterine lining. A thickening would indicate the possibility of cancer. Once, unsure about the results, she had performed an endometrial biopsy to make sure that no cancer cells were present.

But traffic to Dr. Richardson's office kept getting worse and I found it took longer and longer to get there. When my general practitioner close to home offered to take over my gynecological care, I thought it a good idea. She could send me to a specialist if she needed to. Scheduling pelvic ultrasounds became my responsibility.

A few weeks after canceling my regular test, I noticed a telltale streak of blood on my underwear and called my doctor. I knew that this was a symptom that should never be ignored. She immediately referred me to a gynecologist who re-scheduled my test.

<u>May 20, 2020</u>

Like many women who have had children, I was familiar with sonograms. This time, because of my symptom as well as the pandemic, I felt nervous. Covid was surging. The medical facility was all but deserted. Everyone was masked and gloved. I live outside Boston, Massachusetts where standard patient protocol requires medical staff to explain what they plan to do before they do it. The ultrasound technician told me that she was covering a hard plastic "wand" with a condom and lubricating gel, and then inserting it into my vagina. The gel was cold and the wand rigid but not unbearable. I could hear it sending sound waves to the TV monitor it was hooked up to, where a series of black and white images of my uterus appeared.

I knew better than to ask what the sonographer saw. I would have to wait for Dr. Wosu to tell me. She was my new gynecologist, more than a generation younger than me. A few days later, she called to report that my fibroids had remained stable but that the lining of my uterus looked thick. It might be nothing, but could be something. She wanted me to come into her office so she could perform an endometrial biopsy.

"Really?" I asked.

"Really," she said.

That was unwelcome news. Not only because the ultrasound result was unclear and possibly problematic, but also because endometrial biopsies (during which the gynecologist inserts a thin instrument into the uterus through the vagina and cervix, then scrapes off part of the endometrium) are exceedingly painful. I would need a sedative to get through it, therefore someone to drive me. Because of Covid, that person would have to be my husband who would interrogate me about why I needed this additional test and what Dr. Wosu was testing for. I knew she was testing for cancer but I didn't want to tell him before it was necessary. As casually as I was able, I told Patrick that she wanted to take a closer look at the lining of my uterus – did he remember that I had this procedure a few years back? Could he please drive me? In those early days of the pandemic, my anxious husband preferred to drive me everywhere.

June 5, 2020

For years I had been having mammograms and Pap smears and colonoscopies without much drama. I found them uncomfortable, sometimes awkward, often invasive, but they did not leave me feeling shattered. Endometrial biopsies do. Because an endometrial biopsy is so brief – only two or three minutes long – most American doctors do not offer general sedation for the procedure. But however short, this biopsy is excruciating. With my doctor's blessing, I took four Ibuprofens and an Ativan beforehand, but even with Dr. Wosu and her nurse Evelyn Durand trying to be quick, the procedure was as shocking and painful as I remembered. I tried to focus on their faces, tried to breathe deeply and ignore what was happening.

Dr. Uchechi Wosu is a Canadian immigrant of Nigerian descent; her nurse Evelyn, whom I had known for years and whose hand I gripped during the biopsy, is Haitian. Two days earlier, Patrick and I had joined hundreds of our neighbors taking a knee for George Floyd on a mile-long section of our town's main street. As I looked up at their two faces, I thought about the difference between a few minutes of pain in the service of medical help and the seemingly ongoing, unlimited violence against immigrants and America's people of color. Then it was over and I got dressed.

I walked slowly to the parking lot, shaky but determined not to alarm my husband. We had been married for over 35 years and had undergone our share of gynecological issues together.

During the first years, we had been infertile. His parents were sure that I – six years older than Patrick – was the party at fault and let us know it. We hadn't panicked but formed a calm, united front and both underwent testing.

It turned out that Patrick, like a small minority of tall men, had a varicocele – similar to a varicose vein – that raised the temperature in his scrotum, causing a low sperm count and sluggish sperm motility. The operation to seal off the faulty vein required general anesthesia, but he had total trust in his doctors. He had even considered the outpatient surgery so routine that he encouraged me not to miss a day of teaching. I picked him up at the hospital only after he had spent a couple of hours in the recovery room.

Our two miscarriages had further bonded us. One had been early and relatively simple; the other, later, scarier, and requiring a hospital. We now had two grown sons, one grandson and were – we thought – done dealing with our reproductive organs. We were both in excellent health, didn't smoke, didn't drink, ate a Mediterranean diet, worked out, walked our dog three times a day. We lived in Lexington, an historic town in Massachusetts near Boston, surrounded by nature and calm. The danger was Covid. We weren't thinking about cancer.

<u>June 11, 2020</u>

Dr. Wosu delivered the diagnosis over the telephone: *endometrial cancer* – cancer of the lining of the uterus, the most common of gynecological cancers. The others are cervical, ovarian, vulval and vaginal cancer. GYN cancer is not as prevalent as breast cancer and not quite as terrifying as brain or lung or pancreatic cancer, but cancer all the same. She recommended surgery as soon as possible.

I found it impossible to take the diagnosis in.

"Are you sure?" I asked.

"Sure," she replied. I would need surgery and, possibly, chemotherapy and radiation. She asked if I would like her to set up an appointment with AnneKathryn Goodman at Massachusetts General Hospital in Boston, 14 miles away.

I said, "Yes, please."

Patrick had eavesdropped on our conversation and I filled in the details. Neither of us was conscious of having gone onto automatic pilot, shocked numb. We didn't say to each other, *Let's get it out fast before it spreads* though we both probably thought it. We were operating without words or visible emotion, but on the same page. I had never thought about how I would react to a cancer diagnosis. Nor had Patrick. But together we had already gone through several intimate medical procedures and knew how, as a couple, we behaved in medical emergencies. When our younger son was three weeks old and needed a spinal tap, we didn't stop to think: Patrick sped to the hospital with him while I stayed at home with the older one. When my 69-year-old mother had a brain aneurysm and went into a coma, I was the one who had camped out at the hospital while he stayed at home with the kids. The only thought I remember thinking was: *my turn now.*

We called the people we needed to call; made the plans that needed to be made. We felt blessed to be living outside one of the best medical hubs in the world. We didn't even think about a second opinion. Dr. Wosu was so clear about my diagnosis and I trusted her completely.

As it happened, possibly because so many patients were canceling appointments because of Covid, Dr. AnneKathryn Goodman had an opening at Massachusetts General Hospital the following day.

I struggled to keep a sense of control over my life. Like so many people first diagnosed with cancer – did smoking as a teenager cause my lung cancer? – I blamed myself for enabling cancer. I had insisted on pursuing hormone replacement therapy, despite conflicting research studies and the disapproval of some friends. I had been using the low-dose estrogen patch for 15 years because it so significantly improved my sleep, my waning libido, and my overall sense of wellbeing. Was this cancer my fault?

I thought about my casual attitude towards my colds and cuts and bruises that seemed to take longer than usual to heal. Patrick would have called his doctor about each one. I didn't. A year earlier, when a patch of skin on the top of my foot refused to heal many months after a deep scratch, I finally called the dermatologist. She diagnosed skin cancer and operated. Afterwards, I tried to remember to apply sunblock to my skin and stop wearing sandals, but the experience did not pierce my shield-like belief that other people got cancer – not me. And if I had been more vigilant, could I have distinguished between the stomach aches I'd been having since my twenties and the ones I was having now?

Over the years, as friends got sick, I had reacted with what I now recognized as a kind of cancer hubris. Starting in my twenties I knew several women who had breast cancer; I didn't. In high school, one of my best friends had a malignant tumor in her knee and her leg was amputated. That was in the 1960s, when cancer was considered a death sentence. I was asked by her parents and our school administrators to help her recover, and I did both in the immediate aftermath of surgery and during the five years that we waited for a possible recurrence. That experience had significantly shaped my adolescence. My friend had had no recurrence of the disease. That year, however, older people I knew died of cancer, including my beloved godmother who died when I was sixteen.

Back then, few people went public with their disease – as though contracting cancer were shameful or a failure on their part. In the 1970s, when I became a journalism professor, I discovered in the privacy of office hours that some of my students and/or their parents had it: testicular cancer, brain cancer. As an arts journalist reporting for the *New York Times*, I found that celebrities kept their diagnoses even quieter. In 1987, theatrical producer Joseph

Papp worried about being written off and/or losing funding for his theater if he disclosed his diagnosis, at 66, of prostate cancer. As the head of a major New York cultural institution, he was so concerned about being spotted at Sloan-Kettering Hospital that he commuted to Boston's Dana-Farber where Patrick and I found him a specialist. He was treated there until he died in 1991.

Things had changed since then. One of my brothers, like so many other men I knew, had been tracking his rising PSA (prostate specific antigen) for several years before undergoing treatment for prostate cancer. My husband had his PSA tested as part of his annual physical. Because of these routine tests for prostate and breast and colon cancers, cancer *mortality rates* had been decreasing since the 1990s. The *incidence* of cancer, however, was on the rise worldwide. Millions of people, whether they viewed themselves as cancer survivors or disliked the term, now lived with a consciousness of cancer. Compared to Covid in 2020, the disease seemed familiar if not manageable.

The American Cancer Society was predicting 66,570 new cases of cancer of the uterine body in the United States for 2021 and 12,940 deaths. The average age of women when diagnosed was 60. More than 600,000 survivors of the illness are currently living in the U.S. That reassured my husband, a numbers guy. It didn't particularly reassure me but I was still zoned out of any feeling and needing to hear or read the accounts of other women. I also needed to talk through my news with my closest friends.

I called Rochelle, an artist and the mother of three adult children. She herself had not had cancer but, over the past two decades, Rochelle had accompanied a number of women through treatment and death. When I asked if she thought I should tell my sons, Rochelle suggested that it might be better to wait. Why burden them until I knew more? We both knew people who kept illness a tightly guarded secret as well as those who seemed to do nothing but talk about theirs. I wanted to take a middle road. I tried to imagine how telling or not telling my sons about my news would affect them. I didn't want to burden them but I also didn't want them to feel, as one sometimes complained, left out of the loop.

Rochelle and I discussed my family's whereabouts. My 34-year-old son lived in Michigan. He was single, but part of a tight circle of old friends. Over the past year, he had been paying regular sick calls to the mother of one of them as she underwent an arduous course of chemotherapy for pancreatic cancer. She had died a few months earlier – the second mother of his friends to die of cancer. I didn't want him to worry that I was next.

My 32-year-old son and his wife were about to move from New Zealand to Canada with their toddler, despite the pandemic. They were expecting their second child and had lots of other things to worry about. We decided that my two brothers and their wives and children didn't need to be told just yet either. "There's no hurry, is there?" Rochelle asked. At this early stage, only *we* needed to know.

My close friend and I talked about my having what psychologists call a "dissociative" coping style. Patrick had it too. We recognize a painful or dangerous reality, but keep our emotional reactions on hold for later. I think of it not as denial or dissociation exactly, but as a selective attention that shuts overwhelmingly scary things out. That style has worked well for me. When, years ago, my grad school roommate and I were mugged inside our Manhattan apartment, I felt no fear but calmly instructed the burglars as to where our valuables were. When, as a college student, I was caught in the Soviet invasion of Czechoslovakia, I sat down at a typewriter and wrote an eyewitness account of what I observed from the window and heard on the radio. Now, that same psychological defense of dissociation helped Patrick and me think things through. We stuck to our daily routine, walked our dog, ate three meals a day, and tried, each in our own way, to navigate the new landscape.

Patrick is French, born and raised in Paris, where he was educated as an engineer and worked as a technocrat in the Ministry of Industry. Then he was poached by a Boston consulting firm and spent years solving industrial problems for international corporations. For the last decade, he had been an electronic publisher, acquiring, digitizing and proofreading classic books of non-fiction. For the problem of my cancer, he used a consultant's methodology: analyzing, anticipating, and creating strategic scenarios.

As a writer, I worked very differently. Though we both relied on research, I experienced writing as a process of trial and error, almost totally experiential, with little theory involved. For me, it was about asking questions, listening to answers, and sifting through what they meant. I'd been a reporter since the age of 20 and couldn't imagine working without collaborators like my solitary husband. He prefers to work out problems by himself; I enjoy lots of help with mine. One might even say I rely on that help.

After calling Rochelle I stood, socially distanced, telling my news to my next-door neighbor Joelle, a veteran of three different episodes of cancer. I had spent much of her third treatment bringing her fluids to drink and watching several mini-series with her as she moved in and out of sleep. That had been my closest experience of the effect and duration of cancer treatment. She, too, advised me not to tell anyone anything until I knew more, but I decided to write a short email to my family and closest friends. It read:

Just wanted you to be in the loop. I'm meeting tomorrow with MGH oncology surgeon AnneKathryn Goodman to schedule an operation for my endometrial cancer that was just discovered this week. I will know details after tomorrow.

Looking back, I think that writing them the news was an early way to let myself believe it was true.

June 12, 2020

On the day I first met my surgeon, only unaccompanied patients were allowed entry into Massachusetts General Hospital and it would remain that way well into the second year of the pandemic. Parents, partners and significant others were instructed to drive to the roof of a nearby garage, where, we were told, there was fairly good reception that enabled virtual participation in medical consults. We both maintained stoic fronts: a good-bye kiss and Patrick deposited me at Admissions.

Mass General is normally packed, but thousands of patients with heart problems, orthopedic problems, respiratory problems, diabetes, people with routine procedures scheduled as well as people who had been in accidents, were avoiding the hospital. Everyone was terrified of contracting the then-new virus. I was scared too. For weeks I had been sheltering at home with my husband; now, I was acutely aware of sharing breathing space with strangers, and waited in the lobby until I could catch an elevator to the ninth floor alone.

I texted Patrick photos and descriptions of the machines and my surroundings as I went through the preliminaries. The comprehensive check-in: body temperature, blood pressure, oximeter for oxygen level, weight and height. The blood draw. The chest X-Ray. The EKG. The CT scan. The stress test. Each test involved people putting their hands on my body, and leaning their faces within inches of mine. We were all masked, and many of the nurses and technicians were also wearing gloves and face shields. I told myself that these precautions provided an extra layer of protection for them, but they also signaled danger and made me feel an anxiety that I was not yet in touch with about cancer. It did not occur to me that I might "fail" one of these tests.

After two hours of testing, I met my oncologist and surgeon, Dr. AnneKathryn Goodman. While some patients don't have strong feelings about the gender of their doctor, I do. I was pleased and relieved that Dr. Goodman was part of my general demographic: younger than me, but a physician whose quick intelligence reminded me of Martha Richardson. From what I could see behind her large mask and plastic visor, she didn't look anything like the traditional male surgeon in a white lab coat. Skinny as a teenager, her hair a mop of dark curls, AK, as her patients and staff called her, wore blue scrubs and pointy-toed Texan cowboy boots – even in the operating room, her nurses said.

I glimpsed tattoos beneath her sleeves and was glad Patrick could hear her clear voice but not see her. His French idea of a medical specialist was a pompous older man behind a fine desk on a Persian carpet. But Patrick was aware that, despite an informality that would have been inconceivable a generation earlier even in the United States, AK had an impeccable resume for an oncological surgeon. We had looked her up, as we would look up every specialist and every procedure, online. Her bio included: Co-Director of Women's Global Health at Mass General and Director of the Strength and Serenity Global Initiative to End Gender-Based Violence. Several of my Boston friends who worked in human rights knew her professionally. Her idea of vacation, one of her nurses told me, was flying across the world *pro bono* to treat women in refugee camps.

AK had looked me up too. She knew that I was a journalist and seemed comfortable when I took out a pen and notebook, and told her I would be taking notes. Throughout my treatment, I interviewed everyone I met – receptionists, technicians, doctors and nurses, other patients. In my private life, I have known few doctors and was intrigued by the unfamiliar medical universe I had entered. I wrote down information I was given as well as descriptions of anything that struck me as interesting. It was both a long-held habit and journalistic technique. But I soon became aware that it was also a psychological strategy that moved the focus of my attention away from myself and gave me some degree of agency.

After a few minutes of one-on-one, I called and introduced my husband, who was parked on the roof of the hospital garage and would listen in over speakerphone. I had never been as aware of needing a second pair of ears as I was that day. To keep tabs on what was said, to evaluate how the doctor responded to me, to ask the questions that I was too overwhelmed or frightened to ask.

Instead of addressing my biopsy, AK began by asking me what I thought the best therapy might be for Yazidi women in the Middle East who had been raped. She had read online that I had written a couple of books about trauma and recovery. That threw me off and I imagined Patrick on the roof thinking, *Why is she wasting precious time talking about Yazidis instead of Helen's cancer?* I wondered too. To give her a sense of how I thought? To give me a sense of proportion? Some semblance of agency? For her own research? But as I jotted this down, confessing that I knew next to nothing about Yazidi women, I gave her a few bibliographical references about mass psychic trauma, community and cultural interventions.

A doctor friend would later point out that many surgeons are known for ignoring the person in the room and focusing on the problem. By asking me for my opinion about a subject of interest to both of us, my friend pointed out, my doctor was conveying that she saw all of me – not just the part of my body on which she would operate.

After listening to my answer, AK took a meticulously detailed medical history. Maybe she always took her time with new patients, maybe all cancer patients were treated this way in this world-class hospital, maybe it was just a slow day, but I was surprised, and pleasantly reminded of unhurried medical appointments of my childhood, when doctors used to search out data from your face and body instead of from the computer screen.

After my new doctor had my full gynecological history – sexually active since the age of 20 – over 50 years of sex, I realized incredulously as I counted out the years – five pregnancies, two miscarriages, one abortion, two live deliveries, four fibroids, menopause, and 15 years of hormonal replacement therapy. Not atypical, I thought for a woman of my Boomer generation.

"Did HRT cause the cancer?" I asked.

If I was in touch with anything about cancer then, it was with the possibility that I had done something to cause it.

"Unlikely," AK said through her mask and visor. "We can never say 100% but we think it's the grade 1 cancers that are driven by estrogen – not grade 3 like yours." Many women she saw thought that they somehow brought their cancer on themselves, she added. That was maybe a way of maintaining control, but it was not true. What *was* true was that the number of endometrial cancer cases had doubled in the last 20 years, probably because of environmental factors.

There were two key variables pertinent to gynecological cancers, she continued: Grade and Stage. I had missed the information that my cancer was Grade 3.

Stage referred to the phase to which my cancer had progressed, and that information could only be gleaned from surgery. In the case of endometrial cancer, Stage One referred to cancer contained within the body of the uterus. Stage Two referred to cancer that had spread to the cervix. Stage Three meant it had spread to the ovaries and/or adjacent lymph nodes. Stage Four meant it had spread out of the reproductive organs and to other nearby organs, such as the bladder and bowel. Or that it had spread or metastasized via the blood stream or lymphatic system to more distant organs such as the lungs and liver.

Grade, on the other hand, referred to the three classifications of endometrial cancer cells or, as she thought of them, their three possible "personalities." My biopsy showed my tumor as Grade 3, the highest risk category. Its name was "serous "[sic] and it was the most dangerous. It behaved like ovarian cancer and was treated as such.

That scared me. The comedienne Gilda Radner whom I and most of my friends had watched on Saturday Night Live, had died of ovarian cancer in 1989. Unlike the many women I knew who had had breast cancer, received treatment and went back to living their lives, those with ovarian cancer had died.

AK paused to give me time to take this in as well as write it down. I asked no questions and I had made Patrick promise to hold his until after I had asked mine. There was silence from the garage where he, too, was taking notes and trying to take in my situation.

My surgery would be performed laparoscopically, AK continued, using tiny robots. That meant she would be able to operate inside my abdomen and pelvis without making a large incision in the skin. This procedure, also known as keyhole surgery, would perform two functions: therapeutic (it would remove the cancer) and prognostic (it would identify the stage). I would be given general anesthesia and a breathing tube would be inserted to control my breathing during the procedure. Instead of making one long incision, AK would make five small ones in my abdomen. Using small robotic arms and mirrors, and a tiny camera placed in my abdomen, she would cut out my entire uterus and its associated fibroids, fallopian tubes, ovaries, lymph nodes.

This entire "package" would be "delivered" through my vagina. Then the top of the vagina would be folded over, and stitched up like the hem of a dress. The operation would take three to four hours, with an additional three hours recovery time. Unless there were complications, I would go home the same day. Recovery from laparoscopic surgery was typically not painful, AK said, and would most probably not require prescription painkillers once I left the hospital. Just over-the-counter meds. And no heavy lifting for six weeks, as well as no sex, no baths, and no swimming. I wrote it all down.

AK searched what she could see of my face behind my mask and when she thought I was ready, continued. All the material she removed from my abdomen would be analyzed to confirm Grade and Stage. After she read the pathology report, we would have a discussion. Sometimes surgery was all the treatment required. Sometimes more. Chemotherapy was a probability. So was radiation.

It was good that I kept writing because my mind had stopped tracking when she described surgery. It seemed like an awful lot of stuff to take out of my body. Would I feel hollow afterwards? Would my intestines sink to the floor of my pelvis with nothing to hold them in place?

Will I feel empty? I asked AK out loud. I didn't want to use the more graphic term, "disemboweled."

"Nah," she replied. "Think of it as a sock drawer. Uterus, fallopian tubes, ovaries, lymph nodes, cervix – they're all mashed up against your intestines like socks in a drawer. Take out four or five pairs and you don't notice anything missing, do you?"

No, I thought, trying to visualize the inside of what I thought of as my stomach as a sock drawer. But the drawer does look roomier.

Then she asked, "How do you feel about your appendix?"

I started laughing under my mask. I didn't feel one way or other about my appendix, I told her. But my younger brother had recently undergone a scary emergency appendectomy, so I wasn't surprised to hear myself say, "I wouldn't mind if you took it out too."

"Okay," said AK.

My surgeon was, I thought, a unique combination of traditional and contemporary, trained in the latest western medical technology *and* a believer in eastern and alternative medicine including acupuncture, nutrition, exercise and supplements. Starting a B-Complex vitamin daily would serve me well, she said, as would fish oil and chondroitin. Her assistant would be in touch with my surgery date. The best thing I could do during these next two weeks would be to settle any outstanding professional issues, keep up with my exercise, make sure to sleep and eat well. I needed to be in good shape for the operation. And it would be wise to think about how and where I would recuperate from surgery.

Now it was Patrick's turn to ask his questions. He had a tendency to cross-examine doctors and make outrageous demands that he found perfectly normal. I had been mortified a year earlier when he requested that my cataract surgeon walk a straight line just before I was to be wheeled into the OR for the procedure. Without taking offense at my husband's suspicion that he might be drunk and understanding his anxiety, the cataract surgeon had complied. Now, exiled in the garage, Patrick was remarkably restrained. He had already made lists of other surgeons at other hospitals and compiled a spreadsheet of pertinent national and international survival rates for gynecological cancers. He was not out of bounds in his interrogation of AK. By the time we were back home it was all settled. Even though we had agreed not to seek a second opinion, now Patrick felt 100% sure that no second opinion was required.

We are an international family with members and friends on different continents. We didn't want to have a series of conversations about my situation so we put together a group email list and I wrote the first of what would be a series of bulletins to what became over two hundred people. I certainly felt none of the shame that had once hung over cancer patients. I could sense my journalistic skills kick in as I described the new world I had entered. I sensed that writing periodic bulletins would help both Patrick and me get through a year of treatment and recovery.

Jun 12, 2020, 5:28 PM

Dear All:

Please forgive the group email. For those of you that I did not manage to alert by phone, I am sorry to let you know that I have endometrial cancer. My surgeon is AnneKathryn Goodman at Mass General Hospital. This being Boston, she has been vouched for by three of my friends. I am in great hands.

I was given an appointment within three days and my surgery is scheduled for June 25, assuming that I pass a heart stress test. My uterus, fallopian tubes, ovaries and perhaps appendix will be removed. General anesthesia with breathing tube. The surgery should take 3 hours with another 3 hours recovery time. Back home I am encouraged to walk and sit rather than lie around (blood clot danger) and can't have sex, swim or take a bath for six weeks (infection danger), and no heavy lifting (hernias).

After a biopsy of "the package," I will learn how far the cancer has spread.

Friends had urged me to be explicit about my needs so I wrote,

Some of you have asked how you can help. Please hold your questions for the time being. Please send recommendations of your favorite movies and mini-series. For those within driving distance, please bake or cook something. Since Patrick does not cook and I will have trouble shopping and/or organizing meals for the first week. On sunny days, you are urged to come visit outside.

That's the scoop. Tata for now...

Our family (two sons; one daughter-in-law; two brothers; three sisters-in-law, one brother-in-law, seven nieces and nephews) and most of our friends complied with my requests and held most of their questions.

<u>June 15, 2020</u>

I left AK's office with several pages of notes. Once I had time to read them over and compare them with Patrick's notes, I had more questions. I asked them of friends who had long familiarity with the treatment process. Margo, who tended her sister Denise through ovarian cancer until her death; my writing partner Helen, who continues to accompany her wife Donna through years of colon cancer treatment; my friend Susan, diagnosed with leukemia 15 years earlier, who receives chemotherapy every four weeks. Susan was the most matter-of-fact and practical. She said she had learned to acknowledge fear but stay grounded in the present. I should try not to worry about anything until there was something specific to worry about.

I'm lucky not to suffer from anxiety; that's Patrick's department. I, on the other hand, worry about specific impending events, especially the possibility of pain. I worried about the endometrial biopsy and I had been right to worry. Now I worried about the pain of waking up to stitched up wounds. I'm the kind of patient who becomes instantly on guard when doctors use the word "discomfort." I always ask my dentist for novocaine. I remember the labor of childbirth as a long nightmare. My first son took three days to be born. My contractions started and stopped until, on the third day I threatened to throw myself out the hospital window and my docs finally agreed to induce. When I was pregnant with #2, I insisted that my doctor put in my chart: "Drugs on Demand."

I called women I knew who had had laparoscopic surgery to ask about pain. Several had undergone hysterectomies for reasons other than cancer. I interrogated them about how much it hurt. For how long? Had they taken painkillers? When could they bend over? When could they use the stairs? Everyone said that 21st century techniques had transformed surgery. Incisions were small. Recovery was fast. Some of my interviewees had gone to work the next day. They hadn't needed prescription drugs for pain. I didn't believe them.

Although it was not in the forefront of my mind, I was aware that I had, at 73, lived longer than either my parents or my grandparents. All of my grandparents had been murdered during the second world war. None had reached the age of 70. My parents had managed to stay alive during six years of Nazi occupation, through lockdowns, forced separation from their parents, slave labor and near-starvation. Their experiences had seriously impacted their health. They had taught me not to take bad luck personally and to get through difficult situations by focusing on the task or problem directly at hand. Any action was preferable to no action – and certainly preferable to wasting time on feeling. Their way of handling adversity had been in the back of my mind since the start of the pandemic. It was a model I had internalized.

But I was not yet, to my mind, in the thick of it. It was June. I love to garden and I focused on my garden. I also wanted to continue certain other beloved activities and was able to compartmentalize so long as I was absorbed by them. They included reading and writing my share of correspondence, preparing for my weekly Italian language class, my film class and my weekly English tutoring of my Parisian niece. I learned how skilled I was at compartmentalization – even finishing a review of a documentary – *There are No Lions in Tel Aviv* – for an arts magazine. Following Susan's advice not to worry about anything until it became a concrete problem, I decided to take a chance and not cancel a bookstore Zoom reading five days after surgery. Readings gave me pleasure. Why foreclose any pleasure unless I absolutely had to?

June 17, 2020

Since we were having a relatively dry summer, I planned to recuperate outside. I had identified just the right piece of furniture on which to do it: a light wicker *chaise lounge* that I had bought 30 years before and had never used. Now, I thought, Patrick could set it up on our front lawn in the shade. I had never before spent much time sitting on our lawn. Now I planned to do that, bring out my laptop for email and entertainment, watch the birds and chipmunks, and receive friends at a safe distance. I tried out the chaise. It was perfect.

Food was high on my list of significant considerations. Patrick and I had fallen in love over Viennese pastries after we first met at an international conference in Davos. Before Covid, dinner parties were our favorite way of spending time with friends. I shopped and cooked while Patrick did the cleaning up. Now, he would have to learn his way around the supermarket and kitchen, and I would have to learn to plan ahead instead of browsing the aisles for inspiration.

Sex more or less disappeared from our pre-op lives. In the moment and for months afterwards, neither Patrick nor I were interested. I would later read that scheduling of cancer surgery sent some patients of all ages, particularly men with prostate cancer, into a last-call erotic spree. I imagined that both men and women reacted in a wide variety of ways. But the prospect of having my sexual organs removed affected me like the opposite of an aphrodisiac. I had a cancerous tumor inside me; everything was on hold until it came out.

As I made final pre-surgery arrangements, I Zoomed and emailed with people in the UK, Italy, France, the Czech Republic. Covid made some things easier than it would have been otherwise. My friends were all available, at home, on lockdown. Some had contracted the virus. Some had lost family members and jobs and many were distraught. Most had time to write or talk, and being able to connect with them so easily was a blessing at a time when I could have felt very isolated. We compared reactions to the epidemic in their countries and in mine. Everyone talked about how politicians were disregarding science. Everyone talked about the political fragmentation of their society, and how antipathy towards the foreign, immigrants and people of color seemed like a second, concurrent epidemic. I told them how in Massachusetts we, like our neighbors, had Black Lives Matter signs in our yard to honor the lives of so many people who had been murdered in the past few years: Trayvon Martin, Breonna Taylor, Philando Castile, Sandra Bland were only a few of them. Some neighbors had second signs that read: Stop Asian Hate. I was grateful to be living in an environment where I felt safe.

June 25, 2020

There was still no traffic as we drove into the city for my surgery. We were calm and, as I look back on it, trusting. Everything had happened so quickly that I had not had much time to reflect on what, exactly, lay ahead. When my brother was told he needed to treat his prostate cancer, he had already been monitoring his PSA levels for years and had carefully weighed the advantages and drawbacks of treatment options and doctors. We had had no such time.

On the other hand, I was acutely aware of being financially secure, semi-retired and self-employed. Most people receive their cancer diagnoses while immersed in their work schedules and family obligations – most of which are out of their control. Most don't have the time or mental space to focus exclusively on their medical needs. Patrick and I did. We were empty-nesters. Our hospital was half an hour from our home. The costs of treatment would, for the most part, be covered by health insurance. For a cancer patient, my situation was close to ideal.

Did I pray? No. Prayer is not part of my spiritual practice and I did not feel a sudden capacity for it; I find solace immersing myself in art and/or nature. But I gratefully accepted every prayer on my behalf from an assortment of observant Jews, Christians and Muslims, some family members and some friends of friends. I followed AK's instruction to pay attention to keep eating, drinking, and sleeping well, exercising, getting my affairs in order. The morning of my surgery, I lingered in the bathtub and washed my thick, shoulder-length hair, knowing it would soon be a memory. I put on a light loose cotton dress with no waist to pinch me, as I had been advised. I packed a pair of warm socks, a sweater, and my electronics, and we drove to the hospital.

At nine, a good-bye kiss and Patrick drove back home. He planned to distract himself with the all-immersive task of proofreading the eBook he was currently publishing, with breaks to walk Kashu, our Shiba-Inu. His small electronic press had started as a retirement hobby. He had never had much time to read and I had suggested that he digitize classics of narrative non-fiction that had not made the transition from print to electronic media. There were many good books in that category and the process was labor-intensive. You had to select the titles, acquire the electronic rights, digitize them and, because this was not yet a perfect process, proofread every page. Patrick did this with dictation software, listening to every book – including its punctuation – over headphones while correcting pages. It turned out to be excellent work for a person who preferred to work alone and perfect for someone trying to get through a loved one's medical crisis.

How did patients handle the anxious hours in hospital rooms before the internet, I wondered? They had newspapers, magazines, books, radios and television sets, I remembered. They blared from room to room. Today, everything was more private. I brought my electronics and headphones to the hospital and mined the limitless world of the internet. I read emails, Facebook posts, and the latest news headlines, in addition to listening to music until I was given a sedative and I was wheeled into the operating room. It had been decades since I had been in one and since I didn't watch medical shows, it looked unfamiliar to me, like the inside of a spaceship: all stainless steel and constellations of light. Team of astronaut-like figures in masks and face shields. AK said something but I could not make out which one she was. The (male) anesthesiologist began telling me a joke… and I was… out.

I was still out when AK called Patrick and told him surgery had gone well. She had seen nothing of concern, i.e. no obvious metastasis of the tumor, but would not be able to say for certain what lay ahead until after she had the full detailed pathology results. That would be in two weeks. Meanwhile, I was returning to consciousness in a dimly-lit single room, with one of my surgeon's residents asking me if I recognized her. Recognize her? A pre-Covid question, I thought in my own fuzzy state. Surely, she was aware that since she and everyone else on the ward was wearing a mask, patients could barely distinguish gender, let alone recognize a particular face. But I nodded vigorously. She explained that because a previous operation had been delayed, mine had run late, so "in an abundance of caution" I would be spending the night in the hospital.

That came as a relief. I wasn't ready to go home yet. I lay on my back in the hospital bed, watching the reflections of blinking lights and listening to the beeps of machines. Carefully, I tried wiggling my toes. I felt little sensation, and no pain. Someone else popped in to tell me that my anesthetic would not wear off for a while but in another "abundance of caution," I would be given pain medication. My reporter's mind started blinking the warning, "opioid addiction" but I ignored it. "Painkiller" and "abundance of caution" sounded much better to me. I was grateful that my body was all but dead to sensation and that my mind was sailing across time and place with no horizon, no boundaries, no censor.

I reflected for the first time on my missing lady parts.

They had been probed and yanked out of me by strangers. Though I had been drugged unconscious and remembered nothing but the circle of masked faces looking down at me before I conked out, I felt that something momentous had happened. Just as AK had said, I couldn't actually feel anything missing from my body. I felt no sense of loss – just relief at the absence of pain. I checked over and over again, but as one of the dancers sang in *A Chorus Line,* I felt *nothing*.

Surely, I argued to myself, I had to feel *something*. These were my innermost organs removed! My sexual amphitheater. The first cradle of my children. In every culture and era, key symbols of religion, science and myth. I still felt nothing. But a memory I had not thought about in years came to mind.

I was in my twenties, living in Manhattan, and sitting in a doctor's office. I had a burning sensation in my vagina and a yellowish discharge on my underwear. I had called my gynecologist, a kind older man, as I remember. He had examined me, taken a sampling of discharge and left the room to examine it under a microscope as I dressed. Two years earlier, a freelance journalist in search of an assignment, I had been set up to have lunch with a magazine editor. He surprised me by suggesting I write an investigative piece about impotence in American men – a major concern of his readership, he said. I was taken aback. I had no experience with impotence, I told him, and wouldn't feel comfortable interviewing men I didn't know about it. I never took an assignment from him but we struck up a friendship nonetheless, had many more lunches, took trips together. We were sitting in a speeding train holding hands and gazing out at the scenery when I chose to see this moment as a metaphor for the rest of my life and this man as the person with whom I would share it. I moved into his apartment where he edited my writing and introduced me to mind-blowing sex. He also introduced me to his world of newspaper reporters and editors. My brothers had liked him and my mother hoped I'd marry him.

"Are you monogamous?" the doctor asked, when I was sitting in his office.

"Yes," I replied.

He managed to be tactful. "You have trichomoniasis. It's a sexually-transmitted disease. Not serious. Men typically have no symptoms at all. But both of you will need to be treated."

This was not what I should be remembering, I told myself. I should be remembering the two glorious years preceding that, falling in love, travel, our good times. But surgery seemed to have cut loose repressed memory along with my uterus. I remembered trich, ooze, discharge. A punch to the gut. Betrayal. Loss. Grief. Pain. I had been so deeply in love that I thought I would die without knowing I would talk to my beloved that day. For the only time in my life, I stopped eating, stopped feeling, shrank in every way. Mechanically, I went to work and managed to treat my journalism students with care. My colleagues – all men – knew my significant other and told me when they ran into him with another woman. I would never, I vowed, let myself be taken in again.

Why was I thinking about this now? I wondered as I lay in the half-dark, filled with bleeps and blinking machines and shadowy figures beyond the curtains. I couldn't actually feel trauma leaking out of my vagina. But as the title of a best-selling book about trauma suggested, my body had kept the score.

That night, I thought about several women I knew who had had their sexual and reproductive organs removed when they were 30, 40 or 50, younger than I was now. Many had been thrown into immediate menopause, with jarring hormonal consequences. Their psychological and emotional experiences had varied depending on the difficulty of the operation, age and reason for hysterectomy, sexual history, whether they had or had not wanted children – but all had been devastating. But most of them had not been faced with cancer.

I had cancer, I reminded myself. That's why I was in the hospital. My reproductive organs had served me well for the most part. I no longer needed them and was unaware of wishing to hold onto them now that they were obsolete. But I also knew from years of psychotherapy that whatever I thought or felt in the moment would probably change many times.

Cancer treatment with its mix of invasiveness and super-powerful drugs would unleash revelations that, under ordinary circumstances, I would be able to censor even from myself. They emerged sometimes gradually, sometimes in a sudden flash, and it would take me time to realize they were all facets of myself that my body had recorded and stored over years.

June 26, 2020

I woke up on my back in the hospital bed and, cautiously moving to sit up for breakfast, felt something like mild menstrual cramps. My abdomen was swollen, still partially inflated with the gas they had pumped in to facilitate the operation. When I looked down my body, I couldn't see any of the band-aids over the places where AK had made and stitched her five laparoscopic cuts. When a nurse came by to check on me, I asked if I could get up, and discovered that I could swing my legs to the floor with no pain. She disengaged my tubes and wires from my monitors, and I was able to maneuver my IV pole to the bathroom by myself. My numbers were good, she told me when I got back. I could go home.

At noon, Patrick picked me up at the hospital curb. AK had advised him to outfit the front seat of the car with pillows, to drive slowly and to avoid potholes. It was a warm, sunny day with little traffic. Once home, I washed up and changed my clothes. Then I settled onto the chaise that we had positioned under the shade of old oak trees, with a small table beside it and Adirondack chairs for visitors. Patrick brought me tall glasses of Gatorade and the prescribed regimen of medication every three hours, alternating Tylenol with Ibuprofen to minimize stress of the liver and kidneys. *Stay ahead of the pain*, everyone had advised. I found, to my surprise, that I could. I listened to music and dozed.

Surgery had been far less painful than childbirth, I discovered, though its aftermath was very different. After childbirth, there had been a spurt of activity and dozens of new things for Patrick and me both to learn and adjust to. We had also been 30 years younger and I had been so thrilled about everything from my babies' features to the pleasures of breastfeeding that – despite a very sore vagina – I found it hard to sleep. Then, I had been conscious of the enlargement of my life; now, even though I felt no sensation in my vagina, I felt diminished.

I had been given mini-pads to absorb the light but constant trickle of fluid from where my uterus had been. It might last as long as six weeks, I was told. Though they were invisible to others – and I myself forgot about them for hours at a time – the pads reminded me I had been cut every time I used the bathroom.

Bit by bit, I became aware of an almost total absence of my characteristic energy and an equally unusual inability to talk. I'm known for being a talker. Now, talking required too much breath – I had things to say but felt too weak to propel the words out of my body, as though AK had added my diaphragm to the list of other organs to be removed. I didn't want to walk much beyond the five minutes on Patrick's arm every few hours that my surgeon had prescribed. I certainly would not have wanted to go back to work the next day. But I remained dead-set on attending my Zoom Italian class that evening and my Zoom bookstore engagement the next.

Because I couldn't speak or write much, I asked Patrick to take photographs of me that I posted on Facebook – an efficient way of announcing that I was OK to friends around the world. Despite my misgivings about FB, I found it an incomparable way to stay in touch with friends around the world. My urge to visually document my recovery might also have been another way for me to break through dissociation and convince myself that what had happened was real. It was also influenced, I reflected, by my temperament and by changing American cultural conventions around illness.

While many cancer patients kept their treatments quiet in the past and some of my friends still do, I dislike secrets and have never been any good at keeping them. In 2020, I saw no reason to keep my cancer a secret. On the contrary, I thought that documenting my treatment might be helpful to others. I am certain that it gave me a sense of agency in a situation where I had very little. I kept a journal, a medical notebook and a calendar for the same reason.

I also photographed the culinary gifts I received. Chocolates, cookies, pies, cakes. On my first day home, my sister-in-law sent me a surprise brunch package from Zabar's, the Manhattan deli of my childhood. In the photo Patrick took after we unpacked it, I hardly look like I've just had a major operation. My color is good. I still have my good pre-Covid haircut. I look delighted, as though I'm signaling reassurance to myself and my friends: "Look! I'm eating bagels! Don't worry about me!"

I finished everything on my plate in that photo but, apart from the times I sat at the dining room table those first days after surgery, I was either lying in my bed or in my chaise outside. I napped often and, whenever I woke up, tried to drink the liquids Patrick urged on me. He kept me to a strict schedule of pills, fluids and walking every four hours, at first in a very slow circle on the sloping lawn around our home holding my arm. We had been told repeatedly that thromboses – or blood clots – were a serious danger if you did not walk. I would later learn that a friend, operated on for endometrial cancer a few months after me, developed not one but two thromboses in her arm. For the first time in my life, I didn't feel safe walking alone. I realized, with dismay, that I was literally dependent on my husband.

Like many children of immigrants, I was raised to be independent. In what is often a role reversal in immigrant families, I was my parents' ambassador to and interpreter of the new world. After he emigrated from Czechoslovakia to New York, my middle-aged father, a well-known athlete, was often helpless in the city. Since he spoke no English, I served as his translator. My mother, who did speak English, relied on another kind of help. She was often physically ill, and sometimes suicidal. Early on, I became her confidante, household assistant, her cheerer-upper during visits to doctors, hospitals and, above all, during her depressions. As I grew older, I performed that role for my friends and lovers. I was accustomed to being a caretaker. It was only after years of psychotherapy that I had chosen a partner who did not need one but I was still unaccustomed to it.

As soon as he heard my diagnosis, Patrick had embraced the responsibilities of taking care of me. I felt many different ways about this. Grateful but also a little claustrophobic. He behaved like a gymnast's spotter, assessing my balance, anticipating obstacles. He insisted that I have my cell phone beside me at all times. He called me every few minutes when I lay in bed or outside on my chaise and frequently came to check that I was all right. Standing over me with pen and his paper schedule, he brought me my pills and liquids, watched me drink and swallow. In his meticulous way, he recorded the exact time I took my pills and liquids, just as he used to record our infant sons' feeding, burping, sleeping and pooping. I felt infantilized. And while I knew that the discharge trickling out of me was the normal aftermath of surgery – normal, desired, a good thing – I felt as though I was wearing a diaper. I wanted to bathe but was allowed only to shower.

We had brainstormed about bathing in those two weeks before surgery too. To make the shower stall safe, I bought a hot-pink Gorilla Grip mat to keep me – a person accident-prone since childhood – from slipping. But to get in and out of the shower stall there was a step I had to remember. I could not convince Patrick that I could manage it alone and he insisted on monitoring my shower.

I did *not* welcome his surveillance. However, Patrick took this duty as seriously as he did my medication schedule and scrutinized my every move. An "abundance of caution" had become part of our thinking and trumped everything else, including privacy. After some negotiation, Patrick had agreed that I could draw the curtain and that he would not watch as the water ran down my rapidly turning black and blue belly. When I looked down at my body, my breasts hid what he saw. Unless I looked into a mirror, I could avoid almost all of it. I also knew that it was harder for him than for me to look at wounds, particularly at the five bandages on my still-swollen stomach.

The days were already sweat-inducing and every evening, I looked forward to a shower, stepping over the tiled step, planting my feet firmly on the Gorilla Grip mat and standing under a cascade of water. Patrick stood beside the shower stall. Carefully, I ran a bar of soap over and under my torso, then replaced it on its ledge. When the soap bar slid off, I bent over slowly to retrieve it, splaying one hand against the tiled wall, chasing the soap, glad that the sound of running water and the foggy curtain left Patrick oblivious. I engaged in many more such cover-ups as my treatment progressed. While I knew I should be grateful to have such an attentive caretaker, I grew ever more annoyed at being monitored and, on occasion, angry. Maybe I was in denial about how precarious my situation was but our long marriage was predicated on mutual independence. Now mine seemed gone.

From the time I was diagnosed Patrick viewed himself as a watchdog. That first evening his update to friends read:

I picked Helen up at 11:30am today and drove her home very slowly.

She can walk (should walk slowly 3-4 times a day) and do stairs and bend over more or less without any pain but is experiencing a lot of abdominal cramping. That does cause pain and she needs to be medicated every three hours (Ibuprofen alternating with Tylenol). She did not get much sleep last night because of that, so she is dozing off periodically and not doing much talking. She should be much better tomorrow if she gets some sleep tonight.

So please hold off phoning. She has no energy for it right now.

June 29, 2020

During those first weeks, I slept in my son's former bedroom with the door open so that Patrick would be able to hear me if I fell out of bed, or fell as I left my bed, or fell on my way to the bathroom. He dispensed my last pills just before I went to sleep but, despite following every instruction to the letter, I woke up several times during the night. I was afraid to sleep on my stomach or sides, and unaccustomed to sleeping on my back. As AK had said, I felt nothing missing inside. Whenever I awoke, I ran my hands over my swollen belly and remembered that I had had a major operation. The bathroom had a large mirror over the sink and when I disrobed, I now examined my slowly normalizing belly. One of the surgical nurses had covered my stitched-up wounds with five heart-shaped bandages, a whimsical, hopeful gesture unlike the sober descriptions of scarring that I had found on the internet. I took a selfie of those bandages as another document, but showed them only to Rochelle.

Lying on my back alone those early mornings, I felt lucky to be alive and only achy rather than in pain. That was a pleasant surprise. An unpleasant surprise was my unexpected difficulty carrying on a conversation. When Patrick got into bed and snuggled up alongside me, I welcomed his body but found his wish to chat annoying and ultimately exhausting. He asked question after question. Was I in pain? How had I slept? How often had I woken up? Did I need to take my pills?

I tried to answer, but it required energy that I didn't have. As my husband's questions multiplied, I came to prefer the company of our Shiba-Inu Kashu who made no demands and, after checking that I was all right for a minute or two, curled into a ball close by and kept still.

It took some persuasion to convince my spouse that I could manage my morning routine – getting out of bed, brushing my teeth and dressing – by myself. After lingering by my bedside for a few minutes, Patrick went downstairs to make breakfast. I was pleased to see that I could actually do everything I was accustomed to doing and that, if I moved slowly and used the handrail, even going down the stairs posed no problem.

After breakfast, Patrick set up my chaise under the trees and brought me my laptop. I was grateful to be living in a woodsy neighborhood with excellent internet. I could look up at the sky through the leaves of tall trees or browse through the news, my emails and Facebook on my computer. Social media might have serious drawbacks, I thought more than once, but it was a godsend to invalids and convalescents, especially those unable to talk or uninterested in talking. For me, chatting had long been as natural and effortless as breathing; now I became acutely aware of the amount of energy I required to focus on the back-and-forth of conversation, and, even more, to muster the breath and volume to answer questions.

My lack of energy for doing anything surprised me. Was it because my sleep was so erratic? Because my body had taken such a blow? My psyche? I no longer possessed my zest for conversation. I just didn't want it, and realized how annoying my habit of questioning less talkative friends could be. I had for too long been oblivious to their needs, I realized, indulging my own curiosity, oblivious to whether they wished to engage or not. I also had the habit of dispensing unsolicited advice. Now I was on the receiving end and felt ashamed for not understanding earlier how annoying it could be.

For the first time in my life, I had no interest in reading books. I listened to music and movies that were being streamed online. I kept re-watching the movie version of *Hamilton*. Silently, I sang: *In the eye of my hurricane there is quiet*. Like Hamilton, I would write my way out of it.

I *was*, with some preparation, able to attend my Italian class and – five days after surgery – do my bookstore reading. As I applied make-up, I took a careful look at my hair – it would be gone soon and I was glad that a YouTube recording of my reading would preserve how I looked pre-chemo. I managed to get through the hour-long program, but crashed once the adrenaline wore off.

Exhausted for the next few days, I read and reread emails that friends had written in response to Patrick's update. Following my request for their news, they described the various ways they were managing during the pandemic. We were all in emergency mode. Mine was constructed around a rigid schedule of taking my meds, drinking those fluids, walking several times a day, napping and taking in the support of friends and neighbors who visited me on the lawn, keeping a safe medical distance.

July 1, 2020

From: Patrick Mehr

Subject: Helen's surgery – update #5

Today is the 6th day after surgery, and Helen continues to do very well – she is on the computer, sleeps the whole night, regularly walks around the house and the garden, and eats normally.

She still gets tired faster than usual, so she naps during the day. After consulting her brother, she decided to reduce the Ibuprofen and Acetaminophen, but as a result felt some discomfort last night, so she called the surgeon's nurse this morning who instructed her to keep taking all her painkillers until 2 weeks after surgery – "Dr." Epstein thinks she graduated from Med School… ;-)

<u>July 10, 2020</u>

Two weeks post-surgery, we were beginning to feel smug about how well we were managing. Our routine had become as familiar as the route to the hospital and as we drove into Boston, the news on the car radio seemed far more life-threatening than mine. All over the world, more and more people were dying from the pandemic. The President of the United States had withdrawn from the World Health Organization and was holding a large political rally in Florida, currently the leading state in Covid deaths. Many millions more had been rallying to protest the killing of black Americans by police nationwide. The news was so distressing that it distracted both of us from thinking about what my pathology report would reveal and what Dr. Goodman's treatment plan would be.

Significant others were still banned from the hospital, so Patrick dropped me off and drove to the top of the garage. I sanitized my hands, put on a new face mask and headed up to the ninth floor.

It was still desolate up there, with only one other patient in the large waiting room. A technician came out immediately, led me into the labyrinth of corridors and sat me down to take my vital signs. Although I thought I was calm, my blood pressure was through the roof – 180/41 – proof that I was still wildly out of touch with how I actually felt. My temperature was normal. My height and weight had remained the same since prior to surgery, despite those rich, comforting desserts that AK encouraged. Blood oxygen 99%, as measured by an oximeter similar to the one Patrick had purchased at the outbreak of the pandemic. The tech asked me to assess my pain, on a scale from one to ten; I told her that I was no more than a 2.

My tech was pregnant. She and many of her colleagues were young, multi-ethnic immigrants and, as they performed their routine tasks, I asked them where they were from and what their plans were. One question from me and they were pleased to practice their English. For my part, I was glad to focus my attention away from the cold medical instruments and onto their warm faces. I asked where they lived, how they got back and forth from the hospital during the pandemic, what was on their minds. They all felt safe in the hospital, where I was beginning to feel safe too. The thing that worried them most even back at the beginning of the pandemic were the people whom they couldn't avoid sitting or standing beside who refused to wear masks.

One of my former high school classmates, an ER physician, would later tell me how much she learned from my reports of the hospital world. *Let's face it*, she wrote. For the doctor, *the patient walks out the door, and the next problem enters.*

I was determined not to be a problem. I understood that being a hospital patient was being a cog in an enormous and intricate machine. My neighbor Joelle had prepared me for this. Having lost control of my body and my independence, she said, I would now lose control of my time. I had to figure out my own ways of making the best of it and, for me, those turned out to be via electronics. Whenever I went to the hospital, I brought my iPhone, iPad and a charger with me. They were insurance against inevitable delays, mix-ups, mechanical breakdowns, or the emergencies of others. Waiting in a succession of ugly, windowless, claustrophobic exam rooms alone, sometimes for as long as an hour, I developed a new appreciation of good wi-fi.

When Dr. Goodman came in apologizing, as I would discover she almost always did for running late, I took in the sympathetic eyes above her mask, her mop of black curly hair, her lack of a white lab coat, and those startling cowboy boots. I felt lucky that I had a smart, experienced and unconventional surgeon who spoke my language in every sense. If anything, I liked her too much and sometimes forgot I was there on a matter that threatened my life.

She asked how I was feeling and, without thinking, as though we were meeting for a social visit in a café instead of a consulting room, I said, "Fine." Then I took out a pen and the little notebook I had brought along to take notes and ran down how I was doing post-surgery. *No pain. Good appetite. Trouble sleeping at night; napping by day. Walking more.*

I had decided that I didn't want Patrick listening in on my entire consult this time and I was certain that I would not be capable of remembering the answers to what would be a flood of his questions. I tried to get everything AK said down.

Pathology looked great… I scribbled. *Ovaries are perfect, appendix and intestines look fine, lymph nodes negative, no cervical involvement… no sign of travel (metastasis)… but this is a sneaky cancer type that can behave like ovarian cancer… can come back in 20% of women… recommend chemo and a bit of radiation.*

Ovarian cancer and a bit of radiation? That was scary. Somehow I had managed to not remember the close relationship between endometrial and ovarian and fallopian tube cancers. Like almost every other woman I knew, I had seen *Wit*, the play about a middle-aged college English professor with late-stage ovarian cancer undergoing chemo and radiation therapy at the hands of a group of callous male doctors. So, of course, had AK. She was quick to say that cancer treatment had improved considerably in the 30 years since *Wit* was written, as had the knowledge base and bedside manner of most oncologists. "I don't know anyone who behaves like the docs in that play," she said. And, "We're very lucky we caught it when we did."

When AK circled back to ask in detail how I was sleeping, I answered truthfully. "Off and on most of the night. I've never had trouble sleeping before and I've never had to take afternoon naps." When she asked to describe my appetite, I said, "I thought this would be an opportunity to lose some weight but that's not happening." She laughed, said this was not the time to think about losing weight, and gave me a short physical exam before we put my husband on speakerphone. My abdomen was still swollen two weeks after surgery but all but one of the cute heart-shaped bandages had flaked off my skin, leaving the steri-strip stitches beneath them exposed. Gently, AK palpated the flesh below my belly button. Everything felt the way it was supposed to, she said. Time to call my husband. I called Patrick, handed AK my phone, and she launched into a detailed report that immediately swamped my capacity to comprehend it.

I jotted: *Grade 3 (serous)... sneaky cancer... we are very lucky that we caught it when we did... 4-month pregnant uterus, weight 292 grams... stage 1A – means tumor penetrated halfway through the wall of the uterus, 1B is more than halfway through... however microscopic cancer cells can float up from uterus into abdomen and/or settle into lining of the vagina... chemo starts within month... as soon as possible after surgery because it goes everywhere and works well with things that grow quickly... six hours, six cycles every three weeks... could develop neuropathy... Vitamin B complex recommended... Acupuncture good...*

"You're doing great," AK said to me suddenly. I remember the exact tone of her voice in the room. "But the idea is to get it *now.*"

Though I couldn't see Patrick's face, I assumed that he was having an easier time taking it all in. He was accustomed to long, detailed long-distance phone interviews about highly technical matters. Unlike my scribbled notes, his were in neat French handwriting, punctuated by question marks wherever something was not entirely clear. He did not hesitate to ask questions. Though I'm often embarrassed by his interrogations of strangers, this time I was relieved. I didn't have to worry about AK. I was sure she had seen and heard everything under the sun, and she answered Patrick in detail and with extraordinary patience.

Patrick was particularly impressed with her explanation of surgical procedure: she had not evaluated the situation alone but with a board of some 20 specialists, who had discussed my prognosis and determined my treatment. Then she handed me some reading material, apologized that she had a scared, naked, little old lady waiting for her in a nearby room, and said good-bye.

I took the elevator down to street level, got into our car and compared notes with Patrick. We were both relieved that the cancer had been caught at the earliest stage but both worried about its "sneaky" behavior. He had been able to retain far more than I had and that evening, he wrote to our growing listserv:

Update #6

Helen saw her surgeon today, and we heard the results of the pathology report. The news is good: the endometrial cancer has not spread, it's stage 1A.

But her type (what Dr. Goodman calls the "personality") of cancer is "serous" [sic], the most aggressive of 3 kinds. In 20% of cases, microscopic cells of this type may migrate into the abdomen or vagina, so to minimize this risk of cancer reoccurrence, per NCCN guidelines (nccn.org/patients/guidelines/content/PDF/uterine-patient.pdf), Helen will do 6 sessions of chemotherapy over 5 months starting next month, followed by 3 sessions of radiation. Imaging will be used to monitor her.

Her mood is excellent and her recovery from the surgery is going well, but she must take it easy for another 4 weeks, and recurrent fatigue is expected for a few more months. We have total faith in our surgeon and her team and both of us have, uncharacteristically, decided to follow instructions. Please do not be offended if we do not wish to hear your advice! If you have additional questions, please ask me, not Helen, and I can provide more details. We feel extremely fortunate that we are in such good hands and are focused on recovery.

Patrick

His update was as useful for me as for our friends to read. It was true that my mood was excellent and my recovery from surgery was going well. What my husband did not know, because I hid it, was how cognitively overwhelmed I felt, how I could not remember details, or misremembered them, and did not understand their implications.

The chief thing I retained was the information that my hair would begin to fall out soon after I began chemo. Becoming bald suddenly loomed close and real. Unlike having scars on my abdomen, the hair on my head was visible to the world. It would provoke instant reaction, not only from friends but also from anyone walking towards me in the street. I came of age in the Sixties when hair signified more than health, individuality and youth. It expressed who I was. My hair was relatively straight, thick and just above shoulder-length. Like many New England women of my age, I did not color its mix of salt and pepper. But now, as friends offered unsolicited advice about wigs, hats, turbans and scarves, I suddenly wished to become a redhead and began imagining myself with flowing auburn locks. I spent a couple of hours looking up wigs on the internet and began finding wig advertisements on the screen every time I opened my laptop. But I saw nothing that I liked. Then I came across images of Massachusetts Congresswoman Ayanna Pressley.

A few months earlier, Pressley, a wife, mother, and well-regarded local politician, had come out as a bald person.

An African-American known for her elaborate Senegalese braids, Pressley told *Time* magazine that she had decided to stop wearing a wig "to be freed from the secret [of hiding her illness of alopecia], and the shame that that secret carries with it." Congresswoman Pressley said she was speaking primarily to African-American women but she was speaking to me too, and at a critical moment. It took some getting used to her bald look after her beautiful and elaborately styled hair, but I admired the Congresswoman's boldness in going public with her illness. If she could stand up in the House of Representatives with a bald head, why would I hide mine? I thought again about being a redhead and eventually decided on no wig for me.

July 14, 2020

It has not been too bad, I wrote in my journal. I had a book review to finish before chemo began and a few important chores. Patrick had taken over everything else that needed to be done. He was an ideal partner in crisis. I had not spent any time wondering – as some of my friends later asked – whether he would rise to the occasion in sickness as in health. I had married him because he was the most reliable human being I had ever met. We had seen three of our parents through difficult deaths, held hands through two births and two miscarriages. We had traveled well together for 35 years. Getting through cancer seemed like another trip. Our biggest problem, I thought, would be Patrick's anxiety. I would be calm and he would become more and more anxious. But, for now, we were responding in much the same way.

Our two adult children lived too far away to offer help in person. Daniel, an automotive engineer, telephoned every evening from Michigan. Sam, a cognitive psychologist, was in the middle of moving his family from New Zealand to Canada, and texted occasionally. But a virtual parade of friends and neighbors took care of us, bringing delicious meals and great company. As one of them said later, "If you're going to be diagnosed with cancer, the first summer of Covid was a good time." Everyone was working from home. Everyone had time on their hands, no place to go, and was looking to be useful. My friends were pleased to drive to Lexington, have Patrick serve them a latte, and spend an hour under the trees in my shady garden.

I learned a lot about friendship that summer. In elementary school I had memorized the Brownie Scout round: *Make new friends, but keep the old; one is silver and the other gold.* Never having had grandparents, cousins, aunts or uncles, I regarded my friends as surrogate family members and had gone to great lengths to maintain our friendships over long distances, through marriage and divorce, alcoholism and drug addiction. I had rarely thought about which friends would or would not come through in an emergency. Now I found out.

A few disappeared. They had their own histories with cancer or with other serious illness and couldn't handle mine. They were depressed or being driven crazy by politics or the pandemic. I was disappointed but couldn't muster the energy to help with their pain. There were also friends whom I realized I hadn't been enthusiastic about seeing for quite a while. They had always required too much of my energy and, now that it was so limited, I decided not to respond to their calls. But most of my friends showed their devotion and surprised me by showing up again and again. They surprised me with treats, tried not to give unsolicited medical advice, recommended movies to watch and told me their news. Most knew that they should visit for no more than an hour and hold their questions. Many asked only: what would I like to eat? I couldn't keep up with my hydration requirements, so I asked for popsicles – an item I would never have considered ingesting under other circumstances.

July 16, 2020

A patient should never attend a consult alone. For some reason, Patrick and I had not thought it necessary for him to listen in to my pre-chemo consult with AK's head nurse Kathleen Donohue. That was a mistake. As with AK, I retained less than 50% of what I was told and sorely needed Patrick's ears, notes, and memories to supplement my own. I missed some key points and misremembered others.

Katie, as the head nurse was called, had been at Mass General for 40 years and had worked with the surgeon for 26 of them. As earthy as AK was ethereal, Katie seemed to me like a prototypical Bostonian, with the requisite accent and a manner that was kind but bordering on brusque. It would not have occurred to me to examine her shoes. I assumed they'd be sensible and sturdy as Katie herself. I was acutely aware, as I rarely was with AK, that Katie had been answering the same questions in the same way for hundreds of patients concerned about the same basic things. It also crossed my mind that the two of them were like a female version of Don Quixote and Sancho Panza. Already, I felt there were questions I would ask one but not the other.

I took notes again in my little notebook: *July 20th chest port placed... Taxol. Carboplatin... Dose recalculated every time... Steroids before and after.*

"When will my hair start falling out?" I asked Katie. I must have been far less on top of things than I thought because I wrote: *Day 1 falls out Day 17... cold cap can prevent hair loss they say it has a 50 per cent... But freezing cold.*

I would be hooked up to poison and freezing my scalp. I said nothing but thought: not for me.

When would my chemo start?

"As soon as they can get you on the schedule," Katie said.

That was a surprise. I had already forgotten that AK had told me that. It was barely three weeks since my surgery. I still walked slowly and could not get through the day without an afternoon nap. I wasn't allowed to have sex or take a bath for another three weeks.

What should I expect the chemo routine to be like?

"Every 21 days for six cycles, you'll be here most of the day," Katie said. "You come in at 8 am, get your blood work done, wait 45 minutes, then see Dr. Goodman. You go downstairs one floor to the infusion ward around 10 and you're done at 3:30. Most people do well for 2-3 days.

Then fatigue kicks in. Your blood count is usually lowest at days 10 through 12."

I tried to take it in but realized that part of me was saying no.

"You want to avoid crowds. You also need to hydrate a lot. Really a lot. Gatorade. Water. Lots of liquids."

I lagged a minute or so behind Katie: *21 days, six cycles. 8 am check-in. Vital signs protocol... port flushed with saline to prevent infection and blood clots... blood draw to calibrate chemo... also check kidney and liver...*

The business of having to check how my kidneys and liver were holding up during chemo went right by me. I asked, "What's a port?"

Short for port-a-catheter, Katie said. It would serve as the infusion point for the chemo as well as for taking the blood samples she would take every three weeks – sparing me repeated jabs into the veins in my hands and arms. It was a small round plastic device implanted under the skin in the right side of my chest. It was attached to a catheter threaded into a large vein above my heart. The implant involved very minor surgery and stayed in for a year.

"You should get the port this week."

"Do I get sedated?"

"Locally," she said. "Most people have no problem."

Katie explained once again that before every infusion, she would flush out my port with saline solution to keep it clear, and then draw my blood so that the exact dose of chemicals could be calibrated for that day. After my blood was analyzed, AK would come into the examination room to discuss my numbers and how I was responding to treatment. Then I would take the elevator one floor down to the infusion ward. I would be getting two drugs: Taxol and Carboplatin – no matter how hard I tried, I could not remember those two names – both long used to treat GYN cancers. Two nights before chemo, I would start taking a cocktail of meds to inhibit allergic reactions and to prevent nausea. I might develop muscle or joint pain. I might develop peripheral neuropathy. But most people did fine. The hospital volunteers served lunch and snacks and fluids on the ward. Patients brought their electronics. Fatigue was the most common complaint during chemo but she remembered a patient who ran the Boston Marathon after a treatment.

"Are you joking?" It was hard to tell since, of course, Katie was a masked stranger and we had just met.

"The steroids make you feel good the first couple of days. Then the fatigue sets in. And maybe other side effects. There's a 24/7 emergency hotline you can call with problems or questions."

I had enough presence of mind to know that was crucial and wrote down in large letters: *EMERGENCY HOTLINE, 24/7.*

"When do I start treatment?"

"You should be getting a call soon."

Katie finished up by checking that I had written down the emergency line correctly. After the six cycles of chemo ended, she said, I would be coming in every three months and after a while, every six months. Also, I would be having a PET scan on August 24. I remembered my neighbor Joelle saying how little would be in my control and how important it was to thank everyone no matter what they told you. But I didn't feel thankful. I felt overwhelmed by information. I had to dig deep for any positive feeling, let alone appreciation.

Later that day, Joanna called to schedule my port. Katie had said I would be getting a call soon but I hadn't expected it to be *so* soon. I felt rattled.

"I don't even have a start date for chemo," I told her.

"I think you do," Joanna said, rattling me even more. "Let's check. Your first chemo is July 24."

What? How could it be in my online chart without anyone notifying *me*? Or *had* I been notified? Although I was yet to experience true chemo-brain, my memory had already developed major holes. I took a couple of deep breaths and told myself: *You have to fit into their schedule; not the other way around.*

Joanna volunteered that she herself had had a port implanted recently and that it was no big deal. When I asked if she had cancer, Joanna replied: yes, breast cancer. I asked her: had she lost her hair?

Like every other woman I would talk to about cancer, she had a lot to say about hair. I should start looking for a wig right away, she told me. Made with real hair. It would be much more expensive than an artificial wig but well worth the money. She often wore hers – an expensive but very good one – even now that her own hair had grown back. I sat in my chaise under the trees listening to her voice. I had thought briefly about shopping for a wig. I knew Orthodox Jewish women who wore them and looked great. But going to a wig store was out of the question during Covid and after I looked online, I didn't think I would like one, particularly not during the summer.

"Do you mind my asking how old you are?" I asked the scheduler.

Joanna was in her thirties, not much older than my sons. Hair was important to her because she worked in an office and interacted with lots of people. As I listened to her, I was struck again by the variety of women who were contending with cancer. Not only was everyone's diagnosis, and physical and emotional state different, but everyone was in a different work setting and stage of life. Some women were newlyweds; some were new mothers; some were single and dating. And even some of us long-married women, I discovered, were more obsessed by their hair than by their port.

"Very minor surgery," Joanna repeated. "How's next Monday the 20th?"

What could I say but "Of course." But when I got off the phone, I called Susan, my friend who has leukemia, to discuss ports. She didn't have a port and did not remember ever having been offered one. She didn't mind getting infusions in her arms though, after 15 years of them, her veins were getting gnarly. "Maybe," she said, "ports weren't around when I started." Maybe things were handled differently in New York.

I was prescribed a chemical prep for the port implant. I had to scrub my chest for a couple of days with a special antibacterial solution to thwart infection.

Patrick went to the pharmacy to pick up the bottle. Unlike me, he was pleased – not rattled – by the speed and efficacy of the hospital and the multi-purpose efficacy of the port. It was an ingenious piece of medical technology that would facilitate the flow of chemicals into my bloodstream, leaving my hands and arms free to work. But for me the port was an instant symbol and badge of illness. It made chemo (and cancer) real in a way no talking or reading had until then.

July 20, 2020

In the morning, I took my last shower before the implant, scrubbing my neck and the top of my chest with the prescription antibacterial lotion. I tried to persuade myself that this microsurgery was no big deal: thousands of people had pacemakers and heart stents implanted into their bodies; I myself had undergone cataract surgery – three times! – after one operation was unsuccessful. I was walking around with two foreign bodies in my eyes, implants that enabled my vision. But I didn't succeed in convincing myself that the port was a good idea. I knew I would feel it inside me and that Patrick and other people would see the bulge in my skin. There would be no way to pretend it was not there.

Patrick parked in the hospital garage and worked while I changed into a hospital gown, and lay down on a table. Once again, I had a sympathetic woman nurse and doc. I was given a mix of sedatives to help me relax and an anesthetic to block pain. I didn't actually fall asleep but felt pleasantly immobilized, as though I had been placed under a magic spell.

When I returned to full consciousness, I felt a bump where the port had been implanted above my right breast. Unexpectedly, the nurse came over to chat and offer me a pastry and a box of fruit juice. She said I'd soon forget the port was there. She was wrong. When I stood up to leave, I felt the unpleasant sensation of a weight sinking down into the flesh of my right breast. More than anything else, the port would make cancer and chemotherapy impossible to postpone or ignore. From now on it would be ever-present.

When I got home, I decided that the time had come to read *Chemotherapy and You*, the 60-page booklet published by the U.S. National Cancer Institute. I had picked it up on the ninth floor of the hospital, put it on my desk but had not touched it since. "*Rather than read this book from beginning to end*," the wise author advises on the first page, "*look at only those sections you need now. Later you can always read more.*"

I am an avid reader and could not look merely at those sections I needed now. I was in a state of psychic chaos: how should I know what I needed now? I read at my usual breakneck speed: "*Chemotherapy works by stopping or slowing the growth of cancer cells, which grow and divide quickly. But it can also harm healthy cells that divide quickly, such as those that line your mouth and intestines or cause your hair to grow. Damage to healthy cells may cause side effects. Often side effects get better or go away...*" Apparently some did not. I worried which of them would not.

Almost everything I knew about chemotherapy until then came from the play I had mentioned to AK: Margaret Edson's *Wit,* written in the 1990s and made into an HBO movie. The heroine, Vivian Bearing (portrayed by such prominent actors as Emma Thompson and Cynthia Nixon), is a 50-year old college professor diagnosed with stage 4 ovarian cancer. She is a single woman, with no parents, children, or close friends, and she undergoes eight rounds of brutal chemo in almost total isolation. Her male doctors are conducting a clinical trial and appear to be more interested in their research than in Prof. Bearing's wellbeing. So many of her patients had been terrified by

Wit, AK had told me, that she felt it important to explain to them that the treatment portrayed in the play had been vastly improved, that nausea and pain were now well managed, how oncologists were not the sadists depicted, how many were women like herself.

The chemicals I would be given were the same ones that Prof. Bearing got – but the quantities had been "tweaked." They had been used to treat breast, lung, head and neck, and gynecological cancers for nearly three decades. Over those three decades, other drugs had been developed to counter nausea; diarrhea; mouth sores; hair loss; muscle, bone or joint pain; hearing loss; low blood counts (both red and white blood cells); facial flushing; itching; difficulty breathing; and dizziness. I might not experience all these side effects but they were all considered routine.

That would have been scary enough but *Chemotherapy and You* warned that infusions affected people in different ways. "*How you feel depends on how healthy you are before treatment, your type of cancer, how advanced it is, the kind of chemotherapy you are getting, and the dose*."

No one is able to predict how a person will feel during or after chemo, whether they're able to work or not, or for how long. Also, I noted, "*You cannot tell if chemo is working based on its side effects... Side effects have nothing to do with how well chemotherapy is fighting your cancer.*"

All this underscored the extreme uncertainty and unpredictability of chemo. The only thing I didn't have to worry about was how much it would cost. I had Medicare and supplementary health insurance. I wouldn't have financial worries.

In addition to *Chemotherapy and You*, I read two handouts from AK's oncology clinic. *Dietary Goals* emphasized the importance of eating frequently. For the first time in my life, I was urged to eat snacks between meals – not only the usual nutritious fruits and veggies but my choice of sweets. Even more important, as Katie had told me, was drinking: if I could manage to do it, eight ounces of non-caffeinated liquids eight times per day was recommended. Water, juice, soup, milk, smoothies. Failing that, popsicles.

The *Medication Spreadsheet* was the most intimidating. It itemized the drugs and dosage to be taken on the first seven days of each chemo cycle, starting with the night before Chemo Day One: *Dexamethasone* (Decadron); *Senokot* (Senna); *Docusate sodium* (Colace); *Olanzapine* (Zyprexa); and the optional *Ondansetron* (Zofran) and *Lorazepam* (Ativan). These drugs would take care of nausea, constipation and anxiety – apparently the three salient and troublesome reactions to chemotherapy.

Although other cancer patients told me they wanted no one but themselves administering their medication, I was relieved that Patrick took charge of mine. I asked him to buy a colorful pillbox that I had seen in the bathrooms of elderly friends: sunny-yellow compartments for morning pills; blue for evening. In his meticulous way, Patrick took charge of refilling the pillbox every week and checking-up every day on my having taken them. It gave him a sense of control and allowed me one less thing to worry about.

I chose to think as little as possible about tending to my body and, instead, to nourishing my spirit. My nourishment of choice was biographical books and films about people I admired, music and art that lifted my soul. I read all I could find about U.S. Supreme Court Justice Ruth Bader

Ginsburg, and re-watched two films about her life. She was 87 during that summer of 2020, and still working full-time during her fifth course of chemotherapy. I assumed that she had a port in her chest like me and imagined that, if she gave it any thought at all, she thought it small potatoes. Ginsburg had been diagnosed with colon cancer more than 20 years earlier, and had undergone surgery, chemotherapy and radiation. Then she was diagnosed with pancreatic cancer, lung cancer, a second bout of pancreatic cancer and now, she was once again in treatment. She still worked out with her trainer. If she could handle chemo, I thought, so could I.

July 24, 2020

My first day of chemo. Patrick set out my pills with breakfast, checked traffic and figured out when to leave home for hospital. That left me free to pack up a warm hoodie and extra pair of socks, my electronics and charger; a water bottle; and a homemade brownie, all in a cheery yellow tote. A kiss at the curb and he drove back to walk the dog and work, while I texted him my progress through the day: first the flush and blood draw with Katie; then a short consult with AK, still wearing her cowboy boots in the middle of July. She asked me to tell her how I was feeling and what I was expecting. I told her that I was feeling pretty calm but that, as was my habit, I was zoning in and out: in direct contact with my frightening situation for minutes at a time and then not at all. I had prepared for my first infusion by reading what I could of *Chemotherapy and You* and found it helpful, but wondered why chemotherapy had to begin barely four weeks after surgery. Didn't I need more time to recover?

AK reminded me that I had an aggressive grade 3 cancer. It was important to ensure that no microscopic cancer cell had survived the surgery and migrated – into my abdominal cavity or into my vagina. She assured me that it was not too soon for my body to begin chemo. I tried to believe her, but the bottom line was that, finally, I felt really scared. My cancer, she had told me, resembled ovarian cancer and my friend Margo's sister had suffered through ovarian cancer, then chemo and then died. There were so many women who had followed that trajectory. AK gave me a reassuring pat and sent me downstairs. Entering the infusion ward, with its monitors and bags of chemicals hanging from IV poles, I remembered a scene from the movie *The Blind Side*, about the NFL star Michael Oher in his violent, drug-infested childhood home. He had survived by shutting his eyes and ears to what scared him. Semi-consciously, I did the same.

I didn't feel like a chemo patient yet, certainly I didn't think I resembled the other patients in the ward. My hair was still lush and long; my appetite good enough to seriously consider the hospital lunch menu and find it deficient. And I was still recovering from surgery – still wearing mini-pads and trickling discharge.

I addressed the ward as a tourist and took photos to share with Patrick, family and friends: my recliner, the IV pole and chemo bags, the movable food tray, the television set, the striped hospital privacy curtain. I had extended conversations with my nurses and aides.

Courtney – one of the many medics who, since the outbreak of Covid, was touring the country as a traveling nurse – settled me into a beige recliner, and tried to make me feel less frightened by explaining the "tweaks" AK had talked about upstairs. The Taxol and Carboplatin treatment was now prefaced by a "pre-mix" infusion of a steroid, an antacid, an antinausea agent and an antihistamine. Few chemo patients vomited anymore. The Benadryl might even put me to sleep during my infusion. And I would actually feel nothing being injected thanks to my port. I asked if she would take my last pre-chemo photograph, with my still-thick hair. She did. Then, as she hooked me up, I understood another advantage of the port: I could not see the colorless liquid drip from the bag on the IV pole through the thin tube into my chest, or monitor how much was left to go. I was relieved that I was not getting doxorubicin, the lurid red infusion so toxic that breast cancer patients were told to flush twice after using the toilet.

Courtney asked if I generally had cold hands or feet and when I replied that I did, tucked two warm cotton blankets around my legs. Then she plugged my charger into an electrical outlet. I plugged the other end into my iPad, put on headphones, and was soon in my own electronic world. The only disruption to my focus came from a patient on the other side of the curtain who talked incessantly on his cell phone while listening to FOX News. When his voice continued to penetrate into my aural space, I turned up the volume and was pleased to hear him report, "Someone here likes *Hamilton*."

I had chosen to watch the movie of the nearly three-hour musical once again. As I child I attended Broadway matinees with my mother, then listened to recordings of *Peter Pan, My Fair Lady*, *West Side Story* and *Carousel* over and over and over again until I had memorized their every word. My fascination with lyrics was probably the first indication that I would become a writer. As a grown-up, I still liked musicals but rarely took the time to indulge that old desire to listen to them over and over again. This seemed the moment. Time flew by with Lafayette and Washington and Burr, interrupted by aides offering me liquids and old-fashioned Dixie cups of ice cream with the same type of tiny wooden spoon that I remembered from the 1950s. Chemo wasn't hard at all, I texted Patrick and friends; it was almost possible to forget where I was… and why. As the afternoon wore on, patients were wheeled out, the ward grew quieter, and the man listening to FOX left. I thought: I can handle this. It's only six hours a day, only every three weeks. It will all be over before Thanksgiving.

I feel fine, I told Patrick when he picked me up at the curb in the late afternoon. As I had read in *Chemotherapy and You*, I now had very pink, post-infusion cheeks and an abundance of energy, a result of the corticosteroids. When we got home, I took a shower and noticed that my neck and the top of my chest were flushed pink too. The color was flattering and extremely deceptive; I looked healthy and full of beans. Patrick wrote an upbeat update to our email list, signing off in the hope that my treatment would proceed "without a hitch."

<u>July 28, 2020</u>

I had been given a brown paper bag containing pills and instructions. The home drug protocol was clear but complex. No matter how many times I read the instructions, they instantly fled my brain. The night before chemo, some over-the-counter meds for digestion; three tabs of Decadron; then three more the morning of chemo, and then two more mornings. Plus five to seven days of olanzapine (Zyprexa) before bed. All to control the dreaded nausea and possible vomiting. And an entire pillbox of

Ativan (lorazepam) for anxiety. "*You may have a lot of side effects, some, or none at all,*" I had read in *Chemotherapy and You*. There was no way to prepare for what might happen during those first few days after my first chemo session. Every cancer was different. Every patient was different.

I felt pretty much okay that fifth day of Cycle One, only slight aches in the pads of my feet, in my spine, and in the corners of my ribs as I lay in my chaise thanking neighbors for their flowers and cake. I had a bit of "chemo-mouth," cancer sores on my tongue and the inside of my cheeks, and no disorienting symptoms of what was called "chemo brain." I still had my hair. But, I felt exhausted.

I couldn't talk or move much; I listened to music and read my email. I remembered Katie saying that one of her patients had run the Boston Marathon after chemo and now thought she had meant it as a metaphor. Or that maybe patients were wildly different. I was unable to run into the house, let alone a marathon. My energy – boundless as it seemed to some people – was now all but non-existent. There were limits to my interest, my curiosity, my expectations. I felt grateful for phone calls but needed them to be short. Speaking exhausted me. A physician friend emailed: *Talking involves not only having to form the words but enunciating and pushing them out from diaphragm on up using many more muscles and energy.* I ate about half as much as I normally did and found it hard to drink my prescribed eight glasses of liquid per day.

In a short-lived burst of activity, Patrick and I donned plastic ponchos, got out the newly-purchased cordless electric hair clippers our sons had recommended and dragged a stool into the middle of our lawn. Like many other people during Covid, we tried out being barbers. I chose a clipper length of Number Two on the sides, Four on top, halfway to the buzz cut I planned on having just before the days when Katie predicted that my hair would fall out. We took turns being shorn and congratulated ourselves on managing chemo as best we could.

The major problem I was having was my digestion. Typically, my gut was where I lodged my stress. Chemo had irritated my digestive tract even more and was making it hard to both fall asleep and stay asleep. Katie recommended, that in addition to my usual drug cocktail of Decadron, Zofran, and Zyprexa, I add the Ativan routinely prescribed on the ninth floor. It was in my brown bag of medications. That worked, but the next morning, I woke up extremely sluggish. I have little memory of what happened on July 28. I rely on Patrick's update of two days later.

Dear All:

Helen is now back to normal. The faint of heart can stop reading here.

Helen had her first chemo last Friday. Saturday and Sunday were remarkably easy and normal. But she did not sleep well Sunday night, so Monday her oncology team told her that she could add an Ativan to her medications. She did, waking up unusually late on Tuesday. As usual, I went downstairs to make breakfast but when I called Helen, no response. I go upstairs, and find her in an unusual position in bed. I ask what's going on, but no response for what feels like an eternity. She finally says "I felt dizzy while brushing my teeth." She makes it downstairs with my help, sits down, eats one sixth of her slice of toast and egg. I notice she has not had anything to drink and when I give her some Gatorade with seltzer, she spits it out. Now I realize that things are not OK.

I ask her where we live. She can't answer. When I ask "Do we live in California, Oregon or Massachusetts?" she looks at me as if I were speaking Chinese. I call AK Goodman's office; Katie tells me perhaps Helen took Ativan too soon after her other pill, and is having a drug reaction. As I further describe what's going on, Katie says "You have to call 911" which Helen overhears and says "No, I don't want to go to the hospital." Katie says "Helen is in no state to know what must be done. Call 911 right away." Which I do. Ambulance arrives within a few minutes – meanwhile, ever-practical Helen instructs me to put a book and her cellphone in her yellow chemo tote, along with her USB charging cord. Her brain is still working.

I still could walk. Somehow, I had gotten myself from the breakfast table, in and out of a living room chair, and into my office chair.

The ambulance big guys arrive and go into her office where she is sitting at her desk. They run tests ("do this, do that"). Helen says, "I need my phone"; I show her that I have already packed it in her yellow bag. She repeats "I need my phone" and I can see again that something is seriously wrong. I finally realize that perhaps she means her iPad. I run to grab it upstairs, show it to her, and put it into her bag.

I remember a beefy white man standing beside my computer, asking me questions. Then he tied me to a chair and carried me out of my office.

Helen is strapped to a chair by the big men, loaded into the ambulance, and taken to Lahey hospital, seven miles from our home.

I don't remember the ride to the hospital, my arrival, or any of the procedures. The next thing I remember is a private sunlit hospital room on an upper floor.

When I get to Lahey, an emergency MD tells me they are doing tests, and will admit Helen to be observed overnight, so I should go home. Waiting, I can do nothing, not even eat – extremely unusual for me – I call the hospital's emergency room to learn that they are doing an echocardiogram, then a 2nd imaging, then a speech pathologist will see her because of a slight droop in her face and to determine whether she can swallow food; then an MRI. Helen herself calls me from her cellphone at 2:04pm: we speak for 5 minutes, she sounds completely normal, is still downstairs in Emergency and answers my "what's 6 times 8?" correctly and promptly.

Later, I could remember none of this, not even the blood-thinning injection into my stomach. Since Patrick had packed my iPhone as well as iPad, I texted him on and off between procedures, and took photos including a selfie that documented how deceiving appearances can be. My hair had not started to fall out yet. I looked rested and well.

But I could not remember my nurses' or doctors' names, or anything they had said. My memory seemed to have been disabled at the moment that I was carried out of my office by the big burly white man.

At 4:05pm, I call the hospital: Helen is in 6 West, room 1 where I can visit until 6pm. Helen gives me over the phone (again sounding totally herself) a list of 8 things to bring (new underwear, earplugs, eye shade, etc.), items she clearly has thought about herself. Helen patches me in a cellphone call to hear the neurologist Dr. Helenius's report. She is authoritarian, talks very fast with a strong foreign accent, so I barely understand her explain that Helen had "2 small strokes very high up, still a little bit fuzzy in the head, legs weak some, there was a blood clot somewhere else in her body, could be related to the cancer."

I remember Dr. Helenius and her unusual name, that she was extremely bossy and wore a lacy white blouse, at odds both with her martial personality and hospital surroundings. She came from Finland. We dubbed her the Viking.

Dr. Helenius tells us that the MRI shows that Helen had "two embolic strokes." The clot(s) travelled from elsewhere in the body; they checked Helen's heart, arteries, etc., but could not find the clot, which is fine as the clots dissolved naturally and with the blood thinners they gave Helen, including two anticlotting injections in her stomach. Helen "will recover 100% in 2 days to 2 weeks" (she is already 95% herself as far as I can tell); the cancer may have increased the chance of clots because "cancer thickens the blood," but Dr. Helenius was vague on this.

By the time we got home at 6:30 PM, Helen already had a voicemail from AK and an MGH neurologist has been assigned, whom we Zoom with tomorrow at 2:15pm – I am completely amazed at the speed and expertise with which MGH operates! Dr. Helenius had communicated with MGH oncology, and told us – seeming surprised – that Dr. Goodman is "very compassionate."

Helen is back to almost completely normal – only felt a bit dizzy when sitting up from her chair to go walk around the garden this morning.

Patrick

Reading his wrap-up, I realized that neither of us was feeling anywhere near "completely normal." Patrick, however, was invested in thinking so. I realized, even in my own shaky state, that he was exhibiting many of the symptoms of post-traumatic stress. He watched me like a hawk and kept repeating the sequence of events: *You were in such a strange position in bed. You couldn't swallow. You spit out the water I gave you to drink. You said "I want my iPhone," even after I showed you your iPhone! I don't know how I got through it.*

We got through it, I thought in retrospect, by Patrick's disregarding my reluctance to go to the hospital, calling the emergency oncology hotline, trusting Katie and dialing 911, then entrusting my care to a series of people we had never met, the doctors, nurses and technicians at Lahey, the hospital nearest to our home.

The following day we had a virtual consult with neurologist Aneesh Singhal. By all accounts a renowned world authority, Dr. Singhal was a soft-spoken man who had worked in India's largest public hospital. Like AK, he was a social activist and psychologically attuned to shell-shocked patients. During an online consult, he definitively ruled out the possibility of a drug reaction. I had clearly experienced "two small embolic strokes within the context of cancer and chemo." I was very lucky. A year earlier, I would have had to undergo the unpleasant discipline of giving myself twice-daily blood-thinning shots in my stomach such as I had been given in the hospital. But half a year earlier the Caravaggio Study (named after the Italian painter) had demonstrated that people with GYN cancer-associated strokes could replace them with pills.

I zoned in and out as Patrick asked questions about the correlation of cancer and stroke and Dr. Singhal patiently answered them all.

For the next week, Patrick repeated the sequence of traumatic events to anyone who would listen: finding me in bed in a strange position, calling Katie, then 911, my resisting being taken to the hospital. I listened patiently. His recurring intrusive memories of stroke reminded us of the week when our toddler Sam, age three, returned home after a loud fire drill at his day care center. "Big noise," he kept repeating for a week. And for nearly a year afterwards, he would propose, "Let's talk about the fire."

I, on the other hand, had little interest in discussing my episode of embolic strokes. I was focused on getting through my chemo. Once back home, I was focused on my routine of hydrating, taking my pills, snacking as prescribed, napping, entertaining myself with non-taxing, escapist movies, not thinking ahead or back. I had, in little more than a month, experienced a surgery, a chemo cycle and two small strokes. The chemo protocol would proceed. I would not ice skate through my cancer treatment as one of my high school classmates had written to me that she had done. But Patrick and I took two walks every day, slowly, carefully, for 15, then 30 minutes. Everyone said to keep moving. I did.

August 1, 2020

From: Patrick Mehr

Subject: Helen's health – update #9

Dear All:

I am pleased to report that Helen is doing very well, 95% recovered from her 2 strokes of last Tuesday – she is still easily tired, occasionally off balance and once in a while looks for a word as a result of the strokes, in addition to the chemo.

We Zoomed yesterday for almost an hour with Helen's newly assigned MGH neurologist, Dr. Aneesh Singhal (massgeneral.org/doctors/17080/aneesh-singhal) who is calm, clear, brilliant, and enormously reassuring: watch him explain with remarkable clarity on youtube.com/watch?v=mPyP07CLve0 everything one should know about strokes.

Based on this pubmed.ncbi.nlm.nih.gov/32223112 study, out just 3 months ago, Aneesh put Helen on apixaban (or Eliquis eliquis.bmscustomerconnect.com) as a blood thinner, avoiding 2 daily self-injections in the belly. The 2 strokes cannot be, he said, explicitly linked to Helen's endometrial cancer, but cancers are known to thicken the blood, also some time after the cancer has been removed – in Helen's case during surgery 5 weeks ago. And there is no link to the chemo, which will continue as planned.

Thanks to all of you for your concerns about me. Given the givens, I am fine: walking Kashu in the woods is a big help, and my appetite returned immediately after we Zoomed with Aneesh, who I think is quite remarkable. My friend Kalman taught me some breathing exercises and of course it's nice to have Helen back home in wonderful condition. Thanks for all your support.

We really appreciate all your suggestions but we have very clear instructions from the MGH doctors and cannot take in any more information. We also would much prefer reading your emails to speaking over the phone. Helen has to be in total isolation for three days next week when her blood count is the lowest in the chemo cycle, and she would especially welcome your emails and your news then.

Patrick

The weather continued hot and dry and Patrick set up the chaise every day for visits I could have before my three days of recommended isolation. Word of my triple whammy of surgery, chemo, and stroke had spread through my neighborhood and neighbors who had never visited me before now came over. It would be months before I learned about other cancer patients who had subsequent strokes, and read the research specifically linking blood clots to

GYN cancer and its treatment. One of my physician friends whose cancer would be diagnosed just as I was finishing my treatment, developed thrombosis in her arms – twice! – after her infusions. She was put on Eliquis twice a day for the rest of her life, like me.

I lay back and enjoyed hearing my visitors talk. After reading Patrick's update and listening to his recap of the stroke, they were relieved to see that he was still very much himself and that I was a subdued version of myself. Some said that they *preferred* me subdued. I didn't have as much to say as usual but I seemed to be all there. As per Patrick's request, people asked few questions, gave no advice, stayed less than an hour.

My appetite had changed, as both AK and *Chemotherapy and You* had predicted it would. Though Patrick and I had long counted ourselves among the carb-avoidant, I suddenly – with AK's encouragement – began to indulge in carbohydrates: breads, bagels, cookies – all the baked goods that friends brought me. Although I did not experience the predicted metallic taste in my mouth, my culinary desires changed. I no longer could tolerate the sight of sushi or most other fish. I developed a craving for rare roast beef with coleslaw on seeded rye, with a half-sour pickle on the side.

Susan, a friend and harpist who had played in many a hospital waiting room, made it her mission to bring me rare roast beef from a deli in a neighboring town. On occasion, she sat down cross-legged and weeded my garden while telling me her news. Susan had not herself had cancer but was a veteran, having nursed two close friends through years of treatment until their deaths. She was convinced that going through it with an attentive significant other was key. "Diane had no one. Cynthia's husband was not good," she said. “Both of them had pain and nausea during their chemo – you don’t. I hate to say it, but the conditions of your chemo are actually quite pleasant. You’re outside. Patrick makes me a latte. Flowers are blooming. You’re in good spirits. And people like to have a place to go in the middle of Covid.”

My writing partner Helen brought over her specialty *bombe au chocolat,* chocolate-covered fruits, and other caloric treats. Like Susan, she had not had cancer but was a veteran, with the longest and most extensive intimacy with cancer of anyone I knew. Her wife Donna had been diagnosed with colon cancer more than three decades earlier and her experience of doctors had been the opposite of mine: bruising.

Donna had been a young medical technician in a Boston hospital when she discovered blood in her stool, Helen told me, and asked her doctor to order a colon cancer test. The results were negative but Donna continued to experience stomach pain and asked for more tests. “She saw blood in every one of her samples, and yet the doc assured her they were negative. It’s pretty clear that they either didn’t get the results of her test, or chose not to look at them.

“Colon cancer is extremely rare in young people, and Donna was 34 then, too young for anyone to take seriously. They dismissed her as a young woman who could not possibly be sick. She kept making appointments to see them, however, and wasted – as they saw it – their time complaining of pain and ‘claiming’ to have blood in her stool. This went on for over a year. She was repeatedly told by eminent (male) doctors at one of the best hospitals in the world that she must just be having her period. Or she’d drunk red wine. In 1986, she arrived in the ER, violently ill, unable to take a sip of water without projectile vomiting. They chastised her for taking up the ER space and sent her home. Only when she came back a few hours later did a resident override a doctor and suggest they keep her and run some tests. By then, the cancer had spread beyond the colon, into her ovaries and gut, and they had to do emergency surgery, remove everything, put her on a colostomy bag, and when she woke up, tell her she had cancer. And, by the way, the (male) doctor said as he walked out of her room, 'you'll be menopausal.' She was 34 then and wanted nothing more than to have children. She was also alone in the hospital – not because of Covid – but because her partner wasn't a legal relative. Both the homophobia and the misogyny were appalling.

"Donna had a second cancer in 2000 – by then her doc was a woman. And she was a 'known' cancer patient so they took her seriously. It's gut-wrenching just to write this and to remember how women and gay people were treated then."

In many places it is still gut-wrenching, I thought. I did not take my own good fortune with my almost entirely female medical staff for granted. I knew it was the result of years of feminism, as well as timing, geography and the luck of the draw. I was aware of being a white, heterosexual, suburban senior in New England who enjoyed a financial security that my immigrant mother had not had when she was sick. I took nothing for granted. I lay very still in the sunshine, listening to birdsong, breathing deep.

<u>August 5, 2020</u>

A black, imposing medical kit arrived on our doorstep, addressed to me. I had forgotten that, during my post-stroke consult with Dr. Singhal, he had mentioned, in "an abundance of caution," the possibility of my wearing a heart monitor to rule out atrial fibrillation as a cause of my strokes. I had forgotten about it but Patrick hadn't. Now, with dismay, I examined the hard plastic monitor, several adhesive disks to attach to my chest, and their trailing wires. There was no way I would be able to take a bath with all this stuff attached to my body. And where would the hard, rectangular heart monitor go? Next to my port?

"I'm not doing this!" I told Patrick.

"But Dr. Singhal says you need to be monitored."

In what we considered an extended state of emergency, both of us regarded my doctors as infallible. It was psychologically useful to believe that they had all the answers. On an intellectual level, Dr. Singhal had totally blown us away. He was the Co-Chair of Mass General Neurology who had described in great detail treating a TSA employee he recognized from Logan Airport. He had to be under enormous pressure, yet seemed to have time to chat. Trying to walk the line between respect and revolt, I wrote to him:

Dear Dr. Singhal:

Sorry to cause any difficulty but... The heart monitor kit arrived today and I want to delay my using it until after I have completed chemotherapy on November 27. Given all the chemo protocols I am currently following, I do not want to begin using this monitor now. Too much medicalization.

The trade-off in quality of life and possible gain in data re atrial fibrillation is not worth it to me right now.

I feel quite clear about this decision – I did not realize how cumbersome wearing a monitor would be. My husband is anxious that I will have another stroke if I do not wear it. I hope you can reassure him that is unlikely.

Thanks,

Helen Epstein

Much to my relief, he replied,

I had ordered this test (MCOT) just to complete the Stroke evaluation. Regardless of findings, you are going to be on a blood thinner, Apixaban, given the recent GYN diagnosis. The only reason I ordered this test is to determine whether you have atrial fibrillation which may be important if in the future if we decide that you do not need to be on Apixaban. In light of all this, and everything you have undergone, it is totally fine to defer this test indefinitely.

Best regards,

Aneesh Singhal MD

I celebrated.

August 7, 2020

Six weeks after surgery, I could finally take a bath! I sprinkled the Italian bath salts my friend Sue had brought me into the tub, Patrick helped me in and out and I spent half an hour lying in the water, reviewing the past three months as though they were a slideshow.

I still – more than a month later – needed to use mini-pads because the yellow discharge from my surgery was still trickling. It seemed like an awfully long time to me but Katie said it was normal. Little bits of hair had begun to fall from my head and Patrick gave me a buzz cut. I channeled Ayanna Pressley, the Parkland high schoolers, and found an article in *Vogue* magazine that explained how to do it right. Friends worried that, since I was Jewish and many people in my family had been prisoners in Nazi concentration camps, I might find looking at my shaved head in the mirror traumatic. That didn't happen. Patrick did not seem to find my hairlessness upsetting and I suspected that I looked in the mirror far less often than my friends did. I was more concerned that I would shed bits of hair all over the house like our dog.

I was, I realized, not entirely unhappy with being bald. It was August. I disliked all the bother that had to do with hair. Mine had always been a subject of contention between me and my fashionista mother, who for as long as I could remember had greeted me with, "Did you brush your hair today?" instead of "Hello."

I had been born a blonde and she tried to keep me that way with weekly post-shampoo rinses of lemon and chamomile tea. Following 1950s Shirley Temple fashion, my mother also liked to heat up a pair of curling irons and twist my long straight hair into dangling corkscrew curls. When I was about 11, she finally gave in to nature and stopped both rinsing and curling my hair.

I was, for a long time, a compliant daughter. When my mother suggested I get actress Audrey Hepburn's pixie cut, I agreed. But as the Sixties progressed, and I and my friends joined the counterculture, we wanted to look like folksinger Joan Baez, with hair trailing down our backs. Hair not only signified a particular version of femininity but was in the 1960s as in 2020, a political statement.

After the buzz I thought I looked uncharacteristically cool. My scalp certainly felt cool in the August heat, beneath a soft straw hat. It would have been interesting to try out being a redhead, but too much trouble. I found it fun to try out a selection of hand-knit cotton caps and scarves friends chose for me and a multi-colored turban my daughter-in-law sent from Australia. I wore these pieces of headgear inside and out.

Getting to sleep and sleeping through the night continued to be a problem. A friend had brought me CBD *indica* gummies and I tried them a couple of times, but they didn't seem to help. I established a strict sleep protocol: no caffeine after noon, no electronics in the bedroom, A/C and humidifier to counter the hot summer nights, a glass of warm milk or chamomile tea, Aller-tec and melatonin on top of my usual medications, then a chapter of a mildly interesting book. Sometimes even all that didn't keep me asleep for more than five hours and then, during the day, I never knew when fatigue would hit so hard, I would have to lie down. Katie and AK both had urged me to call the 24/7 oncology hotline with any questions, but I hesitated. After my strokes, nothing seemed normal but nothing seemed like an emergency either.

I continued to have an inconsistent ability to retain information. While Patrick googled research studies and had detailed notes from our consults with AK and Dr.

Singhal, I forgot even the key points and numbers. I had never been interested in statistics and that indifference was unchanged by cancer. Unlike Patrick, I did not view doctors or medical literature as the final word. I preferred anecdotal evidence, the personal accounts of individual patients, preferably people I knew.

In none of the handouts we were given, I pointed out to Patrick, had I read anything about strokes or the connection between cancer and blood clots that my neurologist had off-handedly mentioned. Yet I had been told about a friend of a friend with breast cancer in Paris whose stroke had left her partially paralyzed. It sounded suspiciously like what had happened to me, except that I had been lucky and she had not.

My bank of anecdotal evidence was enriched by dozens of women on my high school listserv, who were now also receiving my updates. For six years, I had attended an all-girls school, with some 150 smart resourceful adolescent girls, most of whom had remained in touch. There were several physicians and mental health professionals among us. Given the stats, I guessed that most of us had had direct or indirect experience of cancer and I was soon receiving long emails from those girls – now experienced women – whom I trusted.

My cancer beginning was very scary. Two years ago, my skating was off. I was also constipated. My heart sounded like a washing machine in my ears – swoosh, swoosh, swoosh. I was getting more and more tired out doing very little.

Linnea!!! A tall girl in high school, like me. I remembered being paired with her for basketball in gym. A lawyer now and passionate ice skater.

I met with my doctor. I had lost 10 pounds. I had night sweats. My blood test results were a mess; most troubling was that I only had half my red blood cells.

How confusing. I had been lucky to have had one telling symptom: the streak of blood on my underwear.

A full body PET scan showed lymph nodes throughout my body lit up like a Christmas tree. Stage 4 non-Hodgkins lymphoma was the working diagnosis along with an autoimmune disorder that was killing my red blood cells.

That seemed much worse than my diagnosis.

Well there are about 80 different types of non-Hodgkins lymphoma. Determining the exact type is critical to treatment. After two needle biopsies and a biopsy of a lymph node removed from my neck, the jury was still out. Meanwhile, blood transfusions every two weeks, and then I had another strong infusion when the calcium levels in my blood soared. I was warned that too many of the calcium treatments would disintegrate my lower jaw. Well, so much for vanity...

Yes, I thought. I was lucky that vanity was not one of my personality traits.

Once I started treatment, I had some side effects, BUT I quickly and positively reacted to the treatments. By October, my PET scan showed no cancer anywhere and no swollen lymph nodes!

The science behind lymphoma cures is exploding so my doctor is optimistic that any reoccurrence can be managed. I live each day happy that all fell into place for me medically. I also discovered how many friends and colleagues appeared to support me. That was the silver lining to this whole Cancer ordeal.

That was what I was now discovering.

Finally, very little unglues me now. Worrying is a waste of time. What I have learned is that it is ok to reach out to others for support. That was the hardest lesson for me to learn, but it sure paid off. Ativan made me crazy. I found out that women need a much lower dosage than men. After my loopy experience with Ativan, I only took Melatonin.

Next came an email from Leah. Mysterious Leah often wore dark glasses and I thought her so cool that I rarely dared speak to her. Leah was now a psychotherapist who lived on another continent.

I know your husband said you didn't want advice and there is an occasional bit below, she wrote. *Feel free to delete if you don't want to read further, my feelings will not be hurt.*

That was the kind of cancer candor I had now acquired, I thought.

I had breast cancer, tumor larger than yours but no metastasis, and like you Grade 3 on the biopsy. Had lumpectomy, radiation and chemo. The chemo was optional and different from yours, but I think most of them are a bit of a 'bomb the whole village to get the terrorists' kind of thing.

Breast cancer was the cancer that had struck earliest and most widely in my circle of women friends and former classmates.

Among my cohort, there was huge variation in side effects. I had few initially. I had the ice thing for hair (extraordinarily unpleasant), 95% of which fell out anyway, but my bangs survived which made a difference to me.

Almost every woman I knew told me a version of this. They seemed to forget – or at least not mention – the side effects of pain, nausea, scars, or body changes, but everyone talked about her hair.

Though I didn't have GI tract side effects and always get headaches anyway, I did start after a while to feel very poisoned. I continued going to work but about midway everything began to wear me out. At one point my red blood cell count really dropped and I got a platelet transfusion. Loved it! Wanted more! My red blood cell count had always been on the low side (couldn't give blood when I was menstruating as always on the edge of anemia), just thinking about aerobic exercise increases my heart rate not in a good way…

I stopped reading. It was, as Leah had herself written, too much information at my stage in the process. I would come back to reread it and value it later, after I experienced my own blood count drops.

There were many more emails on our listserv, each in their own way invaluable. Cancer, in 2020, was deeply pervasive in my Boomer generation. Dozens of women I had grown up with had experienced mild or severe bouts of it. Some had had it early, in their 20s, 30s or 40s, and kept it quiet. Some were undergoing treatment in their 50s, 60s or 70s and had reached out in solidarity. That was a source of enormous comfort.

<u>August 14, 2020</u>

The weather had turned very hot and humid. During my daily walks in the woods, trying to comply with athletic Linnea's and AK's urging, I had increased my distance to one mile. Even on my last pre-infusion day, when my blood levels returned to more or less normal, it was a challenge. Followed by Patrick and Kashu, I loved making my way along the shady trails, but wearing a mask was still new then, it steamed up the eyeglasses that I needed to see stones and roots on the ground, and my usual easy 3 mph gait slowed to the slowest of slow motion. Kashu often bounded ahead of me and I had to be careful not to get tangled up in his leash. Patrick tried to stay beside or behind me, to catch me if I teetered. If I tried to walk any faster, I lost my breath and had to stop.

AK and Katie had told me that breathlessness was a common after-effect of chemo, so I was prepared for it. What I was not prepared for were almost daily altercations with unmasked strangers who let their dogs run unleashed, then wanted to tell me how friendly they were, and why it was unnecessary to leash or mask on the narrow trails. Early on in the pandemic, Patrick insisted that we wear masks indoors and out, and became livid when other walkers in the woods insisted on coming up close to argue. Soon I learned to wear a dog whistle and retreat into the bushes to let them go by. I didn't have enough energy for myself, let alone to practice conflict resolution. As I breathed slowly to calm down, I thought about writing an essay about the daily challenges immunocompromised people had to contend with during Covid, a problem that would continue largely unabated.

The last thing I felt like doing when I got home was to fill out the long multiple-choice medical questionnaire that had arrived in my laptop. It was the day before Chemo Two and I wanted to savor my little bit of normalcy. Patrick and I were still processing my stroke, how I had spit up my breakfast, not wanted to go to the ER, how Katie on the emergency line had told Patrick to ignore me, how I had been carried out of my office strapped to a chair. That was hard enough to integrate into my consciousness. I was not yet conscious of having developed the complex phenomenon dubbed "chemo-brain." But, looking back, I see that it was already altering both my mood and cognitive abilities. Although I was abashed to be feeling annoyance when I had the great fortune of being treated at the best hospital around for cancer, I *was* annoyed, petulant and contrary.

Your answers provide your doctor and care team with valuable information to take better care of you, I read. Fat chance! I didn't believe AK or Katie had time for this. My answers would be chewed up by a computer, pored over by statisticians and turned into a research paper that clinicians would never see. It was *easy and confidential,* I read; I just had to choose between the following answers to a question: *Always, Quite a Bit, Sometimes, A Little, Not at All.*

For me, striving for tranquility before my second round of chemo, answering more than 50 multiple choice questions was not easy but a colossal chore. I saw no question about how patients regarded the questionnaire. Instead, it cut right to the chase:

During the past week: Have you had swelling in one or both legs?

Have you felt heaviness in one or both legs?

Have you had pain in lower back and/or pelvis?

When you felt the urge to pass urine, did you have to hurry to get to the toilet?

Have you passed urine frequently?

Have you had leaking of urine?

Have you had pain or a burning feeling when passing water/urinating?

When you felt the urge to move your bowels, did you have to hurry to get to the toilet? Have you had any leakage of stool?

I answered *Not at all* but, of course, wondered whether those symptoms were just ahead of me, maybe in this next cycle of chemo.

Have you been troubled by passing wind?

Have you had cramps in your abdomen?

Have you had bloated feeling in your abdomen?

I wanted to write that I had experienced all these symptoms long before I had been diagnosed with cancer but that was not one of the choices and there was none marked *Other*.

Have you had tingling hands or feet?

Have you had aches or pains in your muscles or joints?

Those questions scared me. I had already heard and read some about neuropathy of the hands and feet, where the nerves in the toes and fingertips are irrevocably damaged by chemotherapy treatment and made permanently numb. The idea of being unable to type or cook properly terrified me, probably more than any other symptom. Maybe because I was hyper-sensitive to this outcome, I imagined I already had neuropathy and answered: *A little.*

Has food and drink tasted differently from usual?

Have you lost any hair?

Have you felt physically less attractive as a result of your disease or treatment?

Have you felt less feminine as a result of your disease or treatment?

During the past 4 weeks, to what extent were you interested in sex?

To what extent were you sexually active?

There was no place to write: post-hysterectomy, chemo and stroke. Did they care? Who knows what hell other patients had gone through in the past 4 weeks. Whether they read English? What their sexual status was? No. We were all one patient mass.

Do you have any trouble taking a long walk?

Do you have any trouble taking a short walk?

Have you had trouble sleeping?

Have you felt weak?

Have you lacked appetite?

Have you felt nauseated?

Have you vomited?

Have you been constipated?

Have you had diarrhea?

Were you tired?

Did pain interfere with your daily activities?

Have you had difficulty concentrating on things, like reading a newspaper or watching television?

Did you feel tense?

Did you worry?

Did you feel irritable?

Did you feel depressed?

Have you had difficulty remembering things?

Has your physical condition or medical treatment interfered with your family life?

Has your physical condition or medical treatment interfered with your social activities?

I closed my laptop, took some deep breaths and tried to focus on why I was so irritable. My brain had been so affected by chemo that it felt onerous to try to distinguish between *Always, Quite a Bit, Sometimes, A Little, Not at All*. Yet it was working well enough to notice that the questionnaire did not inquire about blood clots or stroke – although I had just learned that both were associated with cancer patients. Why not just ask what *we* identified as the worst problems? I would answer: unpredictability. But "How has unpredictability affected you?" was not on the questionnaire.

I began Chemo Two on the morning of August 14 thinking: what else could happen? I was familiar with every step of the routine: Patrick dropped me at the curb. I was given a new mask, used the hand sanitizer, and took the elevator up to Oncology on the ninth floor. After check-in, I waited in the examination room for Katie. She flushed out my port with an injection of saline solution, drew a blood sample, and sent it to the lab. Although I was still disturbed by the weight and bulge of my port, I had come to appreciate that it enabled me to avoid seeing these procedures and left my arms and hands unscathed and easily able to use my laptop and phone. That was all the more important since I might spend an hour or more waiting in the small examination room. After thc labs came back, AK determined my chemo dose, then came in to chat about how I had done during the last cycle. Then I took the elevator downstairs to the infusion ward. Meanwhile Patrick drove home. I texted him progress reports.

When AK came in that morning, she asked only briefly – in what I observed was her habitually calm, kind way – about my strokes. Maybe strokes weren't unusual in her practice or maybe because they were already in our rear view mirror, there was no point spending time discussing them. She had read the notes in my online medical chart, and mostly needed to know whether I felt up to chemo. I said yes – in fact, my body had recovered so quickly that the entire ER episode seemed in the distant past. What I remembered most vividly was my neurological consult with the charming, and impressive Dr. Singhal. When I asked if they had ever met she shook her head, and used another recurrent figure of medical speech: "silos of medical care."

Even at the renowned hospital in which I was being treated, there was little time for in-person cross-disciplinary conversation. Specialists read one another's notes in computerized records and occasionally spoke over the phone: they rarely interacted in person. On the other hand, AK emphasized, she worked closely with Radiation and had an in-person acquaintance with Andrea Russo, who would be my radiation oncologist. Had I made my appointment with Dr. Russo? I would like her. The radiation oncologists, she said, were all "closet physicists" with the kind of personalities associated with that profession, but Andrea was also an empathic doctor, a great clinician.

I laughed, forgetting that we were in an ugly exam room not a café, and that AK was not my friend but my surgeon. It was easier for me to gossip about what Dr. Russo was like than to deal with the prospect of radiation. I had forgotten all about the third block of the treatment – surgery, chemo and something called Brachytherapy – that AK had mentioned at our very first meeting. Suddenly my strokes became a plausible excuse. I couldn't think about radiation at the moment, I told her. I had been through too much for the time being. Couldn't I wait another cycle? Unlike surgery and chemo, the prospect of radiation had terrified me from the start – mushroom clouds, Fukushima – but I felt ashamed to tell that to my heroic surgeon.

All right, she said. I didn't have to start Brachy right away but she asked me to call Dr. Russo's office and schedule my first consult now. I noticed that my surgeon seemed tired and hurried. Coronavirus cases around the globe had topped 17.5 million, with more than a quarter recorded in the United States. It was hot and humid and everyone was worried sick about the political conventions for the upcoming presidential election.

Trying to assess the thin face beneath her face shield and mask, I wondered when AK had had her last vacation. So when she asked me about chemo side effects, I felt self-indulgent complaining. I told her that my biggest problem was sleep. AK advised me to walk and drink more, and to be strict about my "sleep hygiene." Then she sent me downstairs to the infusion ward and I once again began obsessing about radiation. How could I have forgotten that I had to have radiation along with chemo? Did I really? Maybe it could be optional?

Downstairs, I was surprised to learn that traveling nurse Courtney had traveled on. Nisha, who was based at Mass General, was now my primary infusion nurse. Another small jolt. I was having intimate encounters with so many people in such a short space of time that I developed an instant sixth sense about them. When Nisha led me down the infusion ward and stopped before a curtained-off cubicle about the size of a king-sized bed, something about the crisp way she said "Sorry no window," made me like her right away.

There were men and women sitting up or lying down in the infusion ward, some hidden by the curtains, some in full view, old and young, mostly bald, all hooked up to blinking beeping machines, all without a significant other. It was very depressing. If I had felt as though I were ceding my autonomy to Patrick when I took a shower under his surveillance, I ceded it completely to Nisha as she settled me in my hospital gurney, hooked a set of plastic tubes to my port, and wires to the computer. The only way I could manage to control the mix of anger and revulsion at the chemicals that began to drip down into my body was to find a focus of interest elsewhere: to interview my nurse, for example.

Nisha was the thirty-something daughter of Indian immigrants who had grown up in a town next to Lexington. She was a serious student, fascinated by gynecological oncology, taking a graduate degree. I had been a journalism professor for over a decade and sometimes missed the office-hour conversations that came with the job. Nisha reminded me of my grad students and since she came to check on me several times over my four- or five-hour stay, I found her the perfect person to answer the questions I wanted to ask AK but thought too basic for my over-booked surgeon.

As she checked the plastic bags of chemicals against a computer printout and waited for another nurse to crosscheck, Nisha explained the reason I was measured and weighed and my blood was drawn before each infusion. Chemo doses had to be customized from cycle to cycle. The side effects that I reported upstairs to Katie and AK were taken into consideration alongside the blood levels in order to minimize damage to my body. Taxol, Nisha said, was hard on the liver, while Carboplatin was hard on the kidneys. Some patients received smaller doses of chemo but had infusions more frequently. I was getting quite a large dose, she said, and its effects would be cumulative.

This was not pleasant to hear but somehow Nisha explaining it to me made it easier to process.

I would probably find the initial two weeks of each three-week cycle challenging all the way through, Nisha said. And my reactions would become worse with each coming cycle. My blood counts would dip steeply. However, the regimen was designed to allow for a full third week devoted to recovery. I could count on feeling okay – close to normal – during the third week of each cycle. I could plan to do things that needed to be done then. That calendar should give me some sense of control and predictability until I came back for the next infusion.

Like most staff I met, Nisha exhibited great pride in working at Mass General. Its top-of-the-line offerings before the pandemic, she told me, included a spa-like menu of complementary medicine – the in-person services of nutritionists, acupuncturists, massage and music therapists. The pandemic had shut most of it down, she told me that morning, but that week, they had lifted some restrictions and she had noticed the acupuncturist on the ward. I might be able to make an appointment with him. His name was Michael. He gave foot massages as well as acupuncture. Nisha went to tend to other patients and, as luck had it, I soon heard a man's voice asking a patient about ankle pain somewhere beyond the curtains of my cubicle. Hooked up but cut loose from ordinary etiquette, I called out into the ward that when he was done I would like his attention.

Michael, a former playwright, pushed aside the curtains, gave me a mini-treatment, and explained how to reserve an acupuncture appointment for next time. Between Nisha, Michael, the volunteer with the lunch tray, my electronics, a soup and sandwich lunch and the on-offer Dixie cups, my second infusion passed fairly quickly. I was beginning to appreciate the hospital as an extraordinary protected space during the pandemic: a place where people albeit at risk of infection, masked and wearing protective gear, continued to work, interact with patients and colleagues, and live their pre-Covid lives as a vibrant, meaning-filled society.

When Patrick picked me up in the late afternoon, I was in good spirits, flushed pink and as energetic as after Chemo One. The steroid effect, I remembered. *Just like last time.* That little bit of predictability was encouraging. Everything went according to plan. I was able to walk Kashu with Patrick and even to prepare dinner. I enjoyed a novel, same-time-zone Skype with my son and family who had landed in Montreal after a complicated, five-flight journey from New Zealand through several nearly empty airports. When, that evening, I couldn't get to sleep again, I told myself that I was excited, and also that I was under the influence of the nausea-preventing medications. How could I expect to get to sleep? That's why I had Ativan in my brown bag of medications. I took one milligram of Ativan and still couldn't get to sleep. Around 4 am, I took some melatonin.

August 17, 2020

Chemo Two. Day Three. When I tried to get out of bed, I felt groggy, dizzy, and shaky, like a puppet whose puppeteer had let go of his strings. There was something wrong – with my vision, my balance, and my coordination. *This can't be happening again,* I thought. No one has strokes two chemo cycles in a row! I managed to get downstairs clinging to the handrail, and sat down for breakfast trying not to upset Patrick. I took a sip of coffee and was relieved to feel it go down. I took a bite of toast. It went down too. Whatever I was feeling was not another stroke. I could speak intelligibly. I could pass for normal.

Patrick didn't notice anything unusual as I selected my pills from the new dispenser that he had bought and filled: the boxy plastic gizmo marked AM/PM Mon through Sun. I had always felt a hubris about those old people's drug dispensers too and now here I was, relying on them because I couldn't remember what day it was. On the other hand, long unused quotes from Shakespeare or the Bible came to mind: *Oh how the mighty are fallen.*

I was taking what, for me, were an extraordinary number of pills: Zyprexa, Decadron, Zofran, Colace, Eliquis (the blood thinner Dr. Singhal had prescribed), B-complex, Vitamin D, Occuvite, and fish oil. Too many pills had been my thought when I had my strokes.

"Make sure you keep your cell phone next to you," Patrick said as he left to give Kashu his morning walk.

Once the front door slammed, I went online to look up "drug reactions." I had a rudimentary acquaintance with them, having seen friends struggling with cognitive as well as physical issues due to their meds. They had balance problems, problems controlling their hands, problems getting up from chairs and sitting back down. I remembered reading several excellent memoirs by writers who described their drug-induced inability to think straight, type, or write, and their efforts to cover up. I felt some of what they had described. My balance was off. My cognitive function too. But how could I tell what was the cause: chemo, the after-effect of the strokes, my meds?

I had to look no further than one of the pills I took in conjunction with my infusions: Zyprexa, aka olanzapine. Overwhelmed as I was, I had not taken the time to research it and had no idea it was being used "off-label," meaning, "for a condition other than that for which it has been officially approved." Olanzapine, I learned, is "an atypical antipsychotic medication used to treat schizophrenia and manic episodes of bipolar disorder. Side effects of Zyprexa include: akathisia (an inability to sit still), constipation, headache, dizziness, lightheadedness, drowsiness, tiredness, restlessness, weight gain (more likely in teenagers), increased appetite, memory problems, stomach pain or upset, loss of bladder control, back pain, pain in your arms or legs, numbness or tingly feeling, dizziness/low blood pressure, high levels of triglycerides in the blood, high cholesterol, muscle spasms, jerky movements, accidental injury." An incidental finding: Wegmans, Osco and Costco all advertised discount coupons for it.

Hoping I could reach Katie before Patrick got back from walking the dog, I called the emergency hotline.

When I explained what it was I was feeling and my suspecting Zyprexa, she said in her neutral voice, "Stop taking it."

When she asked if I had used up my Ativan, aka lorazepam, (the prescription drug used to treat anxiety and that I had used before my endometrial biopsy) I said no. I was extremely conservative about taking Ativan, I told her. Before cancer and Covid, when I traveled, I used .5 mg on a long airplane flight or to stay asleep in a noisy city. But I was aware that it was addictive: pharmacists would sell you no more than 20 pills at a time. On the Oncology floor, they seemed to dispense Ativan as casually as the infusion floor dispensed those Dixie cups of ice cream. Katie said, again in that neutral tone of voice: "Don't ration it. Some of our patients take one milligram every 6 hours."

That was startling. Maybe in Oncology, patients still suffered such serious nausea or were so desperately anxious, that addiction seemed a secondary concern. But I was concerned. The news was filled with the pandemic of opioid deaths along with Covid deaths. I decided that I would not take any more Zyprexa and I *would* ration my use of Ativan to no more than twice a week if absolutely necessary. I forced myself to drink fluids and flush the drugs that were in my system out of my body.

When Patrick came back, I did not tell him about my conversation with Katie – just asked him to set up my chaise under the trees as usual. I drank an entire 8-ounce glass of liquid as he watched, then brought me another one to sip at while he worked inside. One of my classmates had urged meditation so, after Patrick went back to his publishing, I gazed up through the trees at the sky, focusing on my breathing. But treatment thoughts kept flowing into my brain and I wrote some of them down in my journal. I was as struck by the term "silos of medical care" as I had been by "an abundance of caution." But while the second was probably always a good thing, the first was a disaster for the patient. Apparently, *Oncology knows almost nothing about what's going on in Neurology and vice versa. When I asked who was supposed to be coordinating my care regarding drugs and possible drug interactions the answer was – incredibly – "You!"*

They had to be kidding. I was in no shape to coordinate anything. If Mass General could offer massage therapy, why not a case coordinator trained to bridge those silos? Once again I felt grateful that, at least, I was able to speak English and turned on the coverage of the Democratic convention instead. That did little to improve my mood.

I thought about how critical, impatient and irritable I was becoming, especially with the person closest to me: my partner. I reminded myself that being patient was part of being *a* patient. I had researched and written enough about trauma to be aware that Patrick, by nature more anxious than I, was still shell-shocked by my strokes. He had watched them happen and remembered every step of the process. I remembered almost none of it.

While I just wanted the episode forgotten, he couldn't help watching me like a hawk for a sign of yet another stroke. I had to remind myself that it was normal and necessary for him to keep reminding me to take my pills and keep my cell phone by my side. I was extremely lucky to have him and I should tell him that. I had to be careful about my testiness with other people too. Because of that, and because my energy still tanked after five minutes of talking, it was safer to correspond with friends rather than to have live conversations with them.

I reread some of the emails I had received earlier, when I had felt too overwhelmed by data to take in all they offered. Many of my friends and classmates had written about what had gotten them or people they knew through a similar medical challenge. They all mentioned the need for a good sounding board. Some needed to be alone at home; some needed a companion. Some leaned on their faith or on a trusted minister or rabbi. Others, on their adult children, sisters or brothers. Several mentioned finding solace in their pets.

An unhelpful partner is the worst, Linnea had written. *My husband was in complete denial, because I had never gotten sick before and he could not deal with the notion that I could die. My daughter, who is a clinical psychologist and worked with injured and traumatized soldiers in the VA, was my health care agent. Friends who had experienced cancer (or had a close relative who had) were my best sources of help and support. I try to remove myself from other people's craziness and be kind and nonjudgmental. Help is out there, but I found it very difficult to ask for help.*

I was finding that "help" most often meant women – sisters, daughters, mothers, aunts, housekeepers, best friends of any age – who took the place of a significant other. I had often been one of those people myself. But it was important to let them know you needed help. *If you shut down or self-isolate, the chances of getting that help goes down,* wrote Linnea. *And as you know, a positive attitude fueled with a sense of humor makes a big difference in chances of achieving a complete remission or a complete cure. Hate, anger, despair all raise cortisol and other inflammatory chemicals in your body.*

Audrey, a classmate and now an ER doc in California battling Covid, reminded me to keep a diary of all the things medics like herself didn't know:

Like, who comprises your support systems, what is your home environment like, what happens that scares you, or confuses you? And "how is your family coping?" I don't want to say that we look at each case just as "that lady with endometrial cancer" or "the guy with the prostate cancer," but we don't ever get the blow by blow detail.

I zeroed in on all of that food landing on your doorstep (jealous). It should have occurred to me how little you were capable of indulging in it. As physicians we have a delicate balance of having empathy while making sure that everything goes according to plan – but we don't see the minute to minute reality of how it all plays out. Cancer is always something that will happen to the other guy, not us. So when it does suddenly strike, it can become overwhelming.

I keep cheering you on while wondering about less fortunate people with a similar cancer – no insurance, no support systems, no understanding of why they are lethargic or incoherent. Not to mention lacking the likes of Mass General. You could not be in a better place.

If you write about this the book should be called "A Lucky Woman with Cancer."

PS – The Zyprexa story really threw me. Nasty stuff.

What threw me that morning was an unexpected phone call from Gina, at MGH.

"You have an urgent appointment with Dr. Kozberg in Neurology tomorrow."

Who was Dr. Kozberg? Why was it urgent? Gina had no idea. She was only a scheduler. Patrick was no help either. Each time we were summoned to MGH, he saw it as more evidence of the system's excellence. That night when I could not get to sleep yet again and was reluctant to take Ativan, I took another CBD gummy. Several of my friends used them to sleep and one of them had given me a few.

August 19, 2020

Unexpectedly Patrick was allowed into the consulting room where two female neurologists, Dr. Mariel Kozberg and Dr. Natalia Rost, were waiting for us. I was getting accustomed to my roster of almost all-women doctors and liked it. They seemed less formal than the men and cut to the chase faster. This appointment was, they clarified, merely a routine follow-up. AK had scheduled it the day after I had my strokes but that piece of data, like others, had gotten lost in a flood of information. There was nothing urgent: Dr. Kozberg made clear that after having consulted their boss, brilliant Dr. Singhal, I would find their observations dull. There was really nothing new to report. This appointment was a formality.

She showed us the CT scans of my brain and the area where the strokes had occurred. There was no visual trace of their ever having happened. Then she put me through the standard neurological tests (moving her finger around my head to measure my peripheral vision; tapping and pricking parts of my body, touching parts of my face, watching me walk). Then they asked me questions about post-stroke symptoms. It was hard to sort out, I said, what was stroke-related from what was cancer-related. When I said I was having trouble sleeping and had taken CBD the night before, Dr. Kozberg was displeased. She said that neurologists were seeing strokes in people who used CBD, especially young people. That seemed important. CBD and marijuana were both legal and easily available in Massachusetts, and I wondered why no one in Oncology had mentioned this. Silos again. Dr. Kozberg urged me to take Ativan instead.

August 24, 2020

PET scan day. When AK asked me if I knew what PET (positron emission tomography) scans were, I told her I thought that they were a bit like videos, enabling doctors to measure ongoing processes inside their patients' bodies such as blood flow and chemical changes. I had heard that they were outrageously expensive, used radioactive tracer, and that rich, healthy people sometimes ordered them to ascertain that they had no silent cancer or heart or brain disease. Relatively few hospitals offered the scans, some insurers would not pay for them, and many people questioned the additional exposure to radiation. AK thought PETs were important if you could get them – not a luxury or indulgence. She ordered "baseline" and "post-chemo PETs" in addition to CT scans, in order to verify that cancers she had operated on had not spread. If my insurance balked at covering a PET, she would intervene. I didn't want to waste her time by asking about the many kinds of imaging, so I went online. Researching the procedures I was undergoing, at the time I was having them, proved to be a helpful way of counteracting the many feelings – fear, frustration, confusion – that they engendered.

The least unpleasant, least invasive, and most familiar test I had undergone was ultrasound. Unlike chest or dental X-rays, ultrasound does not use radiation, but transforms sound waves into images. First developed in the mid-1950s in Scotland to detect industrial flaws in ships, ultrasound was soon applied to human bodies. By the end of the 20th century, it was routinely used in maternity clinics throughout the developed world to monitor the development of babies and the uterine environment.

Simple pelvic or abdominal ultrasounds are non-invasive: nothing is inserted into the body. These days, most pregnant women get two or three. They are wired up to a computer monitor; a technician applies a gel to their skin and moves over it with a hard wand-like instrument called a transducer. Transvaginal ultrasound, on the other hand, *is* invasive: the technician inserts a condom-covered transducer into the vagina and manipulates it so as to view as much as possible. I had sometimes found this part physically and psychologically uncomfortable but not painful. Apart from detecting cancer, pelvic ultrasounds are used to locate and examine noncancerous internal growths, ectopic pregnancies and fugitive IUDs, and evaluate pelvic inflammation and fertility problems. Most women I know are relieved to have them.

I found CT or CAT (computerized tomography) scans scarier. They involve lying head facing up on a very narrow padded table and being fed into a tunnel-like imaging machine. Taking images from various angles, CTs provide more detailed information than simple X-rays and are well suited for assessing the extent of internal injuries and bleeding, locating masses and tumors (including cancer), and monitoring the effectiveness of treatments. Relatively quick (many last no more than 10 minutes) the major drawback of CT scans is that they use more radiation than X-rays and immobilize the patient in tight quarters for several minutes, creating difficulties for people with back problems or claustrophobia.

MRIs also involve lying immobile on a narrow table that moves through a rocket-like plastic tube. While these tests do not involve any radiation, they are very noisy, using electromagnets and radio waves. Sometimes the patient is given a dye to drink or take as an injection to make internal structures appear clearer when photographed. Over the years, I had learned to bring my own earplugs.

PET scans were relatively new to me. I remembered having one when I volunteered for an Alzheimer's research study that scanned my brain for plaque. I hadn't had enough plaque to be useful to the study. This time, the combined PET/CT left out my head and scanned the base of my skull to mid-thigh. No prep except to avoid strenuous exercise and eat lightly the day before.

Patrick dropped me off at MGH at 8 am. The machine at MGH looked like I remembered it: like a huge hard plastic life preserver through which the narrow table bearing the patient entered.

This PET was the longest and most elaborate of any imaging procedures I'd had to date, requiring two hours on-site. I changed into a hospital gown and was injected with a radioactive tracer, and then waited 60 minutes for the tracer to be absorbed. Then I was packed onto the padded table that slid into the scanner. I felt at peace and may have dozed off in the dark. The techs watched me from inside a glass booth protected from the radioactivity and left me alone with a panic button for about half an hour while the machine clicked and buzzed and the table slid in and out of the doughnut offering me a view of the stained glass light fixture on the ceiling. After the test, I was told to drink a lot of water to flush the tracer out of my system. We were pleased and relieved to hear that, two months after surgery and one month after I had started chemo, there was no trace of malignancy in my chest, abdomen, or pelvis.

August 30, 2020

Update #12

It's now nine weeks since surgery. I feel more or less recovered from the strokes and drug reaction, and finally accustomed to the portacath. The ever-more-diverse symptoms of chemo, however, continue to make themselves felt. It's like driving on an unfamiliar dirt road in the dark, with sudden dips, bumps and potholes – then, a flat stretch. "At the mercy of our body's vagaries," as a British friend wrote.

I have bursts of energy – usually in the mornings – when I try to weed our overgrown garden and am wiped out after 20 minutes. Then, I lie down on my chaise, sipping from a big glass of water and stare at the birds or try to work on some piece of writing. It's impossible to know what will exhaust me. The one predictable thing is that talking on the phone still does it fast. So please email and text.

I was stunned to read about 43-year-old actor Chadwick Boseman's death today of cancer. He made several films while undergoing chemo and colon surgery.

We just watched him as a very thin Thurgood Marshall. I thought of the many other celebrities who kept their cancer a secret for professional reasons, as many of you have told me that you also did.

Profession, age, temperament and cultural climate all play a role in this. So does how close you think you are to dying. I don't think about dying. I've been told my cancer is a "good" kind, and I choose to believe it. Chronicling the process and sharing it is one of my survival strategies. It draws on my professional skills: observing, describing, structuring, while engaging in adaptive dissociation, as my shrink friends point out.

Luckily, I've had no nausea. But along with chemo fatigue, I do have recurrent neuropathy – toes and soles of feet are okay, then suddenly numb; fingers are mostly fine; hair continues to fall out; itchy skin is new this cycle – but mild compared to last cycle's mouth sores. Appetite still swerving away from fish and anything spicy. I crave bread, bagels, pizza and sweet potato pie.

Be well! Helen

<u>September 2, 2020</u>

According to my calendar, and my radiation oncologist's notes I visited the basement Radiation Oncology suite at 1:30 in the afternoon to meet with Dr. Andrea Russo for the first time, but it seems to have been so traumatic that I have no memory of it whatsoever.

I've also forgotten that I had asked her to send me research studies. They included recurrence rates for gynecology cancer patients who had chemotherapy but not radiation, incidence of post-radiation scarring, damage to the urethra and other side effects of Brachytherapy.

Dr. Russo had immediately sent me two studies.

I don't remember looking at either of them.

<u>September 4, 2020</u>

As Katie drew my blood for Chemo Three, I asked her what patients had told her about Brachy. Katie said, "No patient has complained to me." When AK came in for our pre-infusion catch-up, she looked happy. My PET scan "looked good." As for Brachy, "it's a real snoozer with vanishingly low side effects." And Dr. Russo, "You'll love her." And, confusingly, "The most important thing is chemo. The other stuff is supplementary. Radiation does not improve survival but protects you from vaginal recurrence that can be painful."

What did that mean? I thought this was something that I could discuss with Nisha.

Downstairs, the infusion ward was packed and I was disappointed to find Nisha too busy to discuss anything. My infusion proceeded without incident and I felt confident that this time I'd mastered the drill. You walk out of your infusion with pink cheeks and steroids coursing through your system, and walk a mile that evening. After two days, the steroids wear off. You crash. You force yourself to walk, to drink Gatorade and endless glasses of water to flush the toxins out of your body. You remember the lengthy questionnaire and the meanings of "cumulative fatigue" and "chemo-brain." I was extraordinarily tired. I could not do simple subtraction. I'd go into a room and wonder why I was there. To get *what*? I forgot some words like "pressure cooker" and mixed up others, such as the names of foods I loved like Armenian *lamejun* and the very different Jewish cookie *mandelbrot.* This kind of verbal confusion happened to a lot of people – old and young – who *didn't* have cancer, friends said. But it had not happened to *me* and I felt cognitively as well as physically undermined.

As he had done when I was pregnant, Patrick developed a sympathetic reaction to my symptoms. When a woodpecker woke us up at 6 am, he complained about a "knock-knock" on the windowpane. It was funny and I was pleased to be able to identify the bird to him as a woodpecker but later that morning, when a friend called and asked for directions from the highway to our house, I couldn't tell her and became distressed that I couldn't remember.

I tried to counteract my chemo-brain by writing everything down. I kept notes of my treatment in two journals (one personal, one medical), maintained two calendars, and sent out regular email updates to friends. But there was so much to absorb and so many psychological obstacles to taking it all in! I was relieved to have a fallback in the form of my MGH computerized record that summarized – albeit in medicalese – my case history.

Yet, looking back on it, even all these documents don't add up to a comprehensive picture of my state of being. I divulged different things to different audiences. I minimized, left out, or censored things, like patients often do when talking to their physicians or psychotherapists.

I continued to keep up my schedule of activities no matter what. Treatment affected but did not curtail my writing or attending Italian class, tutoring my Parisian niece in English, performing Zoom readings or watching a schedule of movies for my film class. I rested and rationed my energy. I talked less.

Complaining about aches and pains was usually Patrick's department. But, four months after being diagnosed with cancer during Covid, I was moody, tetchy, even whiny. I still did not worry about dying but I was sick and tired of so many things: having to wear panty liners for that continuing post-surgery discharge; staying hydrated, feeling weak and listless and worried. I kept thinking: what qualifies as enough of an emergency to call the 24/7 oncology hotline? What justifies bothering Katie and the staff? And the recurrent throbbing anxiety: do I really have to undergo Brachytherapy?

Is this an emergency? had come up in the form of a lump on my back about the size of a quarter. My fingers kept returning to it. I tried to see it using mirrors. I asked Patrick to describe it. I took my temperature. Normal but I thought an infection might be developing. It was probably nothing but how would we know? Weighing relative risk, it didn't make sense to go to the ER during Covid.

Had it occurred to me to read through the data from my PET scan that had appeared in my medical chart on August 25 (I only read AK's summary) I would have found reference to a "sebaceous cyst" on the top of my back. I would have recognized the term and known it was not dangerous, but given my chemo-brain, it did not occur to me. I thought, moreover, that the lump seemed to be growing bigger. I began to panic. Should I call the hotline? You never knew who was going to pick up. Katie was on vacation. Was this a big deal or not?

When I finally called, I was put on hold. It was the last week of summer and many staff were on vacation. The man who finally picked up replied in kind when I told him heatedly that I had been waiting for more than 15 minutes. "Don't blame me – I'm just the answering service!" Everyone was working remotely and soon I received a call from an unfamiliar number. When I asked whether my bump constituted an emergency or not, the nurse told me the only way to have it examined was in an Emergency Room. It was my call. I had once watched our vet lance a similar lump on the back of our dog Kashu. I asked Patrick to lance the cyst on my back. It healed.

September 6, 2020

Did I have to do Brachytherapy? That question kept creeping back to mind: the closest I came to fear during the entire steeplechase of cancer treatment. Although I was then only partially aware of it, three rounds of chemotherapy had deeply affected not only my blood counts but my cognitive functioning, my emotional state, and my judgment. I stood before the bathroom mirror in the morning brushing my teeth and stared incredulously at my bald pate which still had a few stray wisps of hair. This was me now. Maybe I should have gotten a wig. I had not yet scheduled my radiation consult with Dr. Russo though AK had twice told me to. I couldn't think about it and, for once, Patrick didn't push me. For whatever reason, he wasn't sure about radiation either.

Part of my state of mind was that in the middle of chemo, I simply could not bear to think about another kind of poison. Had I been able to be my usual counterphobic, intrepid self, I would at least have researched Brachy. But fear made that impossible. My brain stopped working and instead of learning the details of this highly localized, short course of radiation, I conflated it not only with general radiation but with radioactive fallout from nuclear war and nuclear disasters like Three Mile Island, Chernobyl and Fukushima Daiichi.

Brachy, I understood only *after* I had undergone the treatment, differs from other radiation in that it places radioactive material directly inside or next to the area that needs to be zapped. The technique is widely used in prostate cancer, cervical cancer, gall bladder, lung, rectal, eye and vaginal cancer. But during Chemo Three, I simply could not tolerate knowing that.

I think about radiation every time I fly and every time I go to the dentist. If they drape you in a lead apron when you have X-rays, how can radiation be a good thing? Like many school children during the Cold War, I had participated in air-raid drills and knew where the nearest fallout shelter was. I read books about the effects of radioactive fallout.

One of those books, *Hiroshima* by John Hersey, was a classic of American journalism. In a stellar example of unconscious acting out, I had chosen to review a new book about the post-war journalists who had gone to Hiroshima in 1945 to investigate what had happened. Hersey had questioned the bombing and exposed the U.S. coverup of radiation illness among Hiroshima survivors. I managed not to notice that I was reading and writing about his investigations into the effects of radiation while refusing to do it myself.

When I reread Patrick's update #6, I see why AK viewed radiation as part of my treatment. *"In 20% of cases,"* he had quoted her saying to us, *"microscopic cells of the grade 3 serous type may migrate into the abdomen or vagina, so to minimize this risk of cancer reoccurrence, per NCCN guidelines (nccn.org/patients/guidelines/content/PDF/uterine-patient.pdf), Helen will do 6 sessions of chemotherapy and 3 of radiation."*

I had no recollection of AK saying that. Forgetting is a key survival skill in cancer treatment. So is refusing information. I had never clicked on the NCCN (National Comprehensive Cancer Network) link. I had never even asked Patrick to summarize what he had read and, in my journals, made no mention of the third part of treatment looming ahead.

Several kinds of fear of damage arose in my mind: scarring inside my abdomen; damage to my digestive and urinary tracts; seeding of secondary cancers; shrinkage of my vagina. I don't remember what finally made me schedule my Radiation Oncology appointment or who I saw in the ominous basement that day. What I do recall was a virtual Zoom consult with three Radiation Oncology staff – Dr. Andrea Russo, her nurse Yoshie Sawin; and, unexpectedly, a resident fellow. The resident was first up. This pleasant young man had been tasked with taking my case history, starting from day of diagnosis. I was instantly annoyed and uncooperative.

Why was I, four months into treatment, being asked to go over the chronology of my surgery, strokes, and chemo with the resident? So that he could get some practice? I was being treated in a teaching hospital, generally a great boon for the patient. Students had been present all along and I hadn't gotten annoyed. I even had gone out of my way to put them at their ease. But before, the topic had not been radiating my last remaining lady part.

Five minutes into the interview, I had decided that I would cancel the three Brachy sessions scheduled for me the following week. But I was too much of a coward to tell him. I didn't want to seem non-compliant or sexist or since he was a South Asian man – racist. After Dr. Russo took over and described the actual procedure of inserting a kind of lead tampon into my vagina and then zapping it, I was almost catatonic. By the time she handed me over to her nurse and explained how I would receive a dilator to stretch my vagina every other night for a few weeks and then once a week for the rest of my life, I decided to email as soon as I got home.

Dear Dr. Russo:

After our meeting and also with Dr. Goodman, I've decided to postpone brachytherapy until the end of chemo. I have a history of UTIs and intestinal troubles and don't think that this would be a good time to add to them. Also, I would like to read more statistics on the efficacy of brachy after surgery + chemo before committing to brachy. I'm not sure that the balance of caution and side effects works for me. But that is all for future conversation. So I am canceling the appointments scheduled for September and will revisit this in November when I'm finished with chemo.

All best,
Helen

She, like AK, did not argue with me. She wrote back:

I will ask my office to cancel the upcoming appointments and schedule a follow up in November to discuss further. Good luck with chemotherapy.

Best,

Andrea

September 10, 2020

Although I had told my docs that I was only postponing – not refusing – I spent the week googling "refusing treatment." Patrick continued, uncharacteristically, to keep quiet, possibly because he didn't realize how serious I was about refusing Brachy. "It was your body," he later said. "You had to decide what was best for you." My docs thought so too. When I later asked AK directly, she said, "In my spoiled life, refusing part of treatment doesn't happen frequently. But when it does, I try to be present and listen to people sort it out. Bullying a patient into something that doesn't feel right is damaging. And if you don't have free will, what do you have?"

I told very few friends that I was thinking about opting out of radiation. I knew that some of my friends virtually boycotted western medicine – I even had one friend who refused to be vaccinated against Covid. Others were skeptical of alternative medicine. I had no interest in or energy for arguments. After three episodes of cancer as a "perfect" patient, my neighbor Joelle told me that she believed in doing whatever her doctors told her to do, so I didn't solicit her opinion either.

Given the long history of cancer treatment, there are relatively few studies about patients who refuse a treatment. They often leave their docs and become unavailable for follow-up research. Yet googling "refusing treatment" yielded nearly 76,000,000 hits and I started reading about a very large group of "difficult" and non-compliant patients in the haphazard way that I tell friends and journalism students never to do.

Much of what I found about refusal of treatment was directed at physicians, like this note from the Vermont Ethics Network:

Every competent adult has the right to refuse unwanted medical treatment. This is part of the right of every individual to choose what will be done to their own body, and it applies even when refusing treatment means that the person may die. A person might decide against having a recommended treatment for religious reasons, because it is too risky or expensive, or because there is little chance it will get them back to a quality of life they could accept, or because treatments are only going to prolong the dying process.

It is not the patient's job to simply "go along" with what is being recommended. Rather, the patient's job is to consider all the options and decide what is best for him or her. What is most important from the medical point of view may not be most important from the patient's point of view, because goals and values may differ. As long as the patient has been given all the relevant information about his or her treatment options and knows the risks and benefits of each option, including the risks and benefits of turning down treatment, the patient's wishes come first.

I was more interested in reading case histories and found an interesting one about an Israeli woman – a sister Boomer – who refused treatment after surgery for breast cancer in 1997. It was written by a family physician who had been so impressed with her that he subsequently went on to develop a distinguished international practice in integrative oncology.

Keywords: Patient-doctor communication, Cancer care, Complementary medicine, Refusing treatment, Declining cancer treatment, Alternative medicine.

During my years of consulting cancer patients and families, Dr. Moshe Frenkel wrote in the *Oncologist*, *I noticed an increasing number of patients who declined conventional cancer treatment, a phenomenon that piqued my curiosity but somehow was not acknowledged by my colleagues, other than to mention that they had another "difficult patient."*

Suzanna, he continued, had been in her mid 40s, when she underwent surgery, which confirmed stage 3B breast cancer with metastasis, and was advised to begin chemo as soon as possible. *She came to me distressed and ambivalent about undergoing chemotherapy. During our prolonged and charged discussion, she suddenly asked me a question I had never heard from any of my patients. She asked me to look through the medical literature and determine her chances for recovery if she received chemotherapy. With my limited knowledge of oncology at the time, I assumed that the survival rate would be around 80%.*

After consulting the literature, however, I was surprised to find that, given her advanced disease stage and the chemotherapeutic agents available at that time, her chances for survival would be only 32%.

When I shared this bad news with her, she didn't seem too upset. In fact, she asked me to do her another favor: to search the medical literature again and see what her chances for survival would be without chemotherapy. With both sadness and conviction, I told her, "You will die." Still, she urged me not to jump to conclusions, but to take a second look.

So, I dove into the research once more. To my surprise, during that time, when the Internet and PubMed were relatively new, finding the answer to her question in the current medical literature was not easy.

Finally, after spending a few hours in the local medical library, I unearthed a relevant article that estimated the survival rate of women with diseases at the same stage who did not receive chemotherapy. It was 26%.

At that point, Suzanna firmly said: "Look, chemotherapy would add only 6% to my survival rate. But I would lose my hair, which is so precious to me, it would affect my social interactions, and I would suffer nausea and vomiting. In fact, the oncologist gave me a list of side effects two pages long! I've decided that I am willing to risk losing the theoretical 6% advantage chemotherapy would give me. Chemo would destroy my quality of life. I am not doing it."

I told her she was making a great mistake, and I tried to change her mind... Her oncologist, an experienced physician, informed her that she had 6 months to live if she did not follow his treatment recommendations, and if that was her decision, there was no reason for her to continue to see him. Nonetheless, she decided against chemotherapy and began trying a wide variety of alternative and complementary therapies that she heard about from other cancer patients...

The number of patients who make this decision is not very well known, but the number appears substantial enough to warrant close attention. Studies have reported rates of less than 1% for patients who refused all conventional treatment and 3%-19% for patients who refused chemotherapy partially or completely. We tend to think that refusing therapy leads to a poorer quality of life as the disease progresses without treatment. Interestingly, that might not be the case.

A study that evaluated the quality of life of 140 cancer patients who had refused, discontinued, or completed chemotherapy revealed that the quality of life of patients who refused or discontinued chemotherapy was no different than that of patients who completed treatment.

In my interactions with patients who seek advice about complementary therapy options, I occasionally meet patients who have actually decided to decline treatment. Some have shared their decision process to refuse treatment, partially or completely, but most have not shared this decision with their treating physician. More commonly, during their search for second or third opinions, patients do not return to any of their original physicians for treatment and are lost to follow-up. Patients are looking for a physician, to share their decision with a trusted professional who is willing to listen to their account of their painful journey...

As to Suzanna, to my initial astonishment, she thrived. In 2007, she published a book with an inspiring title: Six Months to Live, Ten Years Later.

This was a highly unusual and moving testimonial by a physician whose advice had been rejected, I thought. Far more persuasive than other rejections of treatment I had read or heard. Another sister Boomer I had known, then a young mother of two daughters, had also been diagnosed with breast cancer. She had started but then rejected chemotherapy. But unlike Suzanna, she had died. I wanted to hear Suzanna's own version of how she had lived – but I didn't want to track her down and find out that maybe she had died. It wasn't until a year later that I found her email online, wrote to her and learned, as Suzanna wrote me, that she was "alive and kicking," still practicing integrative therapy, and writing another book.

I was not entirely surprised. Members of my Central European family had long used homeopathic and herbal medicine for their ailments and my own mother gave us charcoal pills when we had the runs. Her aunt Grete Schutz had been one of Vienna's first female pharmacists, when drugs were often still dispensed as herbs. She began every day by standing on her head, practicing yoga and ingesting a large quantity of vitamin and mineral supplements until her death at 94. Grete's sister Lily also took supplements and played the piano till she died as the City of Berkeley's Oldest Citizen at 106. MGH was open to integrative medicine. But, unlike Suzanna who was certain that she did not want either chemo or radiation, I felt ambivalent. I needed to consult with someone I trusted, before the internet and medical silos, someone like the GPs of my childhood.

September 14, 2020

Over the course of my life, I've had dozens of doctors and saw them in many different kinds of medical settings. When I was growing up in New York City in the 1950s, our elderly Czech doctor still made house calls. After he retired, I graduated to the practice of one of three short Viennese sisters who practiced out of a large apartment on Central Park West. One of the sisters kept house; the second kept the records; the doctor conducted long conversations and physical exams and gave unequivocal instructions.

When I went to college in Israel, I first encountered socialized medicine and more unequivocal instructions. I was told I had five rather than four wisdom teeth, one was on top of number four. My case was unusual enough to warrant a class and, during extraction at Hadassah Hospital, a surgeon I had never met before cracked jokes to the group, ignoring the fact that though anesthetized, I was conscious. At the same community-oriented hospital, getting birth control pills, I lay in stirrups in a suite of examining rooms with open doors, hearing the doctor talk about gynecological issues with a wide variety of Israeli Arabs and Jews, as well as international tourists. Pregnant in Massachusetts when health maintenance organizations were popular, I was seen in a private room but by a group of obstetricians. I accepted the fact that I couldn't choose who would deliver my babies.

After cancer surgery, I no longer felt resigned to a revolving door of doctors. I needed one principal care physician who was trustworthy and relatively easy to reach. I found Dr. Devasena Balasubramaniam, aka Dr. Bala.

To find a good doctor anywhere in the world these days is a blessing. My last general physician, fed up with time management strictures, had left to work in a boutique practice. Dr. Bala was recommended by a friend who had grown up in a Communist country, where one still locates a competent doctor through the grapevine and then bribes him or her with liquor or dollars. She had adapted this custom to Boston by donating to her doctor's practice. Dr. Bala was yet another immigrant. She had been an ophthalmologist in India, performing open-air cataract surgeries by the hundreds. She exuded serenity and I imagined her patients opening their eyes after surgery and conjuring an angel. Though grounded in traditional Western medicine, she – like AK – encouraged acupuncture, meditation and applying daily warm compresses to soothe tired eyes.

I knew that Dr. Bala could not spend boutique time with me or coordinate the various silos of my treatment. But I asked if we could have a video consult and it turned out to be even more helpful than I had hoped. Even over Zoom and through the disorienting fog of third-cycle chemo-brain, Dr. Bala was able to reassure me about the temporary nature of specific symptoms such as breathlessness and chest pains, and assuage my amorphous dread of radiation. I spoke openly about what I was feeling and she helped me clarify my options.

I didn't read her notes at the time but, looking back at them a year later, I see how extraordinarily helpful it was simply to say what I felt to a good listener, to be carefully listened to, and have my words repeated back to me, along with the reactions of a well-informed physician.

Dr. Bala's notes read in part:

She is in her third cycle of chemotherapy and it is getting harder. This week was quite difficult. She had called the nurse hotline at the oncology department on Thursday, and they sent her to MGH for a blood draw. By the time she had her blood draw on Friday she was back to normal. Some of her levels continue to remain low. After this, her symptoms recurred over the weekend including some chest pain. She has declined radiation therapy now as she felt it was too much. She is aware that there are many side effects of radiation on the urinary tract and the intestinal tract and also causes vaginal atrophy. She is also aware that in order to examine the shrunken vagina, the Gyn dilate it twice a week for two years; she is stressed about the same. She also has concerns about vaginal scarring. Hence, she deferred the treatment for now and the oncologist agreed to her wishes. She had asked the Gyn if this treatment increases life expectancy but was informed that it did not.

- *I explained that chemotherapy is potent.*
- *I agree with holding off radiation therapy for now if needed.*
- *Discussed that the main aim of the intervention is to treat cancer and minimize the risk for recurrence.*
- *At 73 years, if the amount of radiations affects quality of life then the quantity of life is not important to the patient.*

And about those recurring and worrisome chest pains, which I had also not mentioned to anyone else:

Reports atypical chest pain over the weekend which was waxing and waning. Describes pain like sensation of an "impinged nerve" in the region of fifth or sixth intercostal junction. Has twinges of pain which happen when she is lying in bed in the mornings. Inquires what she should tell her husband given he wants to take her to ER if she reports pain and how to differentiate between costochondritis and something serious. She did have similar symptoms a long time ago for which she had been to the ER for two days. After coming back from ER, her PCP told her that pain was likely due to costochondritis. Inquires if there are ways to evaluate the heart without going to the ER.

- *Costochondritis could be due to chemotherapy.*
- *Discussed the nature and associated clinical manifestation of costochondritis pain (musculoskeletal pain) and heart related pain. We may consider reevaluation for the heart if pain lasts for five minutes longer at a stretch.*
- *Recommended alternate ice and heat compress. Benefits reviewed.*
- *Recommended to use topical rubs like Biofreeze, Arnica gel, and Tiger Balm to reduce discomfort.*
- *Discussed that she may have relief when she lies on her back and extends her ribcage may relieve the spot.*
- *Suggested to explain to her husband about costochondritis, not worrisome as her investigation results were normal, and she would agree to see the ER if pain lasts longer.*
- *We may consider proceeding to the emergency room if her pain due to costochondritis worsens. Discussed*

the characteristics of pain which may prompt her to go to ER.

- *Discussed symptoms which may prompt her to go to ER for evaluation.*

The old journalism prof in me particularly enjoyed her summary assessment:

No acute distress, well-kempt.

Normal appearance.

Speaking in full sentences. No observed coughing, wheezing or distress.

Awake and oriented, normal speech.

Behavior appropriate. Normal mood, affect, thought and cognition.

September 18, 2020

Long before I was diagnosed with cancer, a friend sent me a kind of diagnostic chart, assessing the value and maintenance of friends. I thought it was crass. I come from a very small family, and friends play an outsized role in my life. I had read Cicero and Emerson on friendship and often thought of writing a book of my own. While delight in another's being, complementary personalities, common interests, shared histories are obvious reasons for some friendships, the reasons for others are mysterious, and the costs of maintenance change over time. I usually go above and beyond to keep friendships alive, through marriages and divorces, over long distances, political differences and addictions. I didn't need a "friendship diagnostic chart."

During Chemo Three, that chart floated to mind. It sorted friends according to Value and Maintenance, as in "Low Value/Low Maintenance" – not great but not requiring much investment – or "High Value/High Maintenance" – requiring a great deal of attentiveness but worth it or "Low Value/High Maintenance" – best to dump him or her – or "High Value/Low Maintenance" the best of all worlds.

Henry James once advised writers to be people "on whom nothing is lost." Forced to be passive, watching friends who came to visit, reading their emails or listening to them on the phone, I observed a great deal about my friends. Some whom I'd considered less than reliable, turned out to be stalwart. Others, who I thought would be wonderful, were not. The terms Value and Maintenance became pertinent. I even found myself exercising friendship triage. I stopped engaging with friends who didn't nourish me; I discovered those who did. By Chemo Cycle Three, I had no slack to cut anyone, no resources to humor or console or excuse. I was usually a reliable support person – but I had lost the capacity.

Happily, most of my people had signed up for the long haul. My two American brothers and two sisters-in-law kept in constant careful touch. My observant Jewish French family prayed for me. Many friends continued emailing, recommending music, movies and livestreams from all over the world. The locals kept on bringing chocolate. Others brought good company though they were themselves ill or had sick partners, difficult work or children with special needs. Because of the pandemic, those children were now home full-time. Everyone was exhausted, yet they came through for me again and again.

Other friends, however, had disappeared completely or I wished they would disappear. I had no energy at all for casual acquaintances. Through my books and my speaking engagements, I had over the years met hundreds of people, who liked to write to me, who sent me manuscripts to edit or blurb, or films to view. That was out of the question now. It felt weird to do but I learned to play the cancer card, and reply, *"I'm sure you didn't know that I've been ill and cannot..."* That usually ended the correspondence. But sometimes, it only encouraged more.

So sorry to hear this news, I heard back from a couple of filmmakers. *We hope with all our heart that you recover quickly and continue with your productive life. We also had a very difficult Covid year. In April last year our daughter, Jenny, died of colon cancer after fighting for 3 and a half years. Our older brother Salomon, died of brain cancer last October, and another brother, Rafael, died of a surgery on the heart last February. Hugs and warm regards...*

I'm sure that they meant well but their email felt like an imposition. I didn't want to read about cancer deaths, not from friends, not from strangers. Except one. That evening, news broke that Supreme Court Justice Ruth Bader Ginsburg died after 20 years of being treated for cancer. She was 87 years old and a role model for me. In addition to living a full life, she had made it through colon cancer in 1999, pancreatic cancer in 2009, lung cancer in 2018, pancreatic cancer again in 2019, working, enjoying her family and friends, going to the opera, and exercising till the end. She focused on what she loved and kept going as long as she could. There were two films recently made about her. I watched them again and again.

September 26, 2020

I fell going up the stairs.

The previous day, Day One of Chemo Four, all had gone as expected. The techs took my vital signs. Everything was as usual: pulse, temp, blood pressure, weight. Katie flushed my port and did my blood draw. But AK was on vacation, *her* version of vacation, Katie said in that neutral voice of hers – volunteering in camps for asylum seekers on the Mexican border. I tried not to smile and didn't try to probe what she, Katie, thought of this. I thought, as usual, that my surgeon was a heroine.

Taking AK's place today and giving me a physical exam was Nurse Practitioner Maria Avila-Wallace. AK had talked Maria up and I could see why. Awesomely competent, she was yet another smart woman on my medical team. Maria was from Puerto Rico and spoke very much like people in my childhood neighborhood on the West Side of Manhattan. As she placed my feet in stirrups and peered into my vagina, she mentioned that she could see one of my stitches that had not dissolved after surgery. Even though it was now three months since surgery. It should disappear soon, she said. Sometimes the stitches took longer than expected to dissolve.

Who knows whether it was that childhood connection or something about Maria herself or maybe, that day, I had reached the limits of trying to behave like the perfect patient. When she asked how I was doing, I told her the whole truth. I was exhausted, occasionally breathless, dizzy, slightly incontinent, and worried about my short-term memory, muscle weakness and the numbness developing in the tips of my hands and feet. I also told her that I worried how radiation might scar my urinary and digestive tracts and shrivel my vagina. I told her I had been molested as a child and had reached the limit of my tolerating assault of my vagina. I told her the truth: that I didn't want to *defer* Brachy; I wanted to *refuse* it.

Maria was another deep listener. She didn't interrupt me, answered some of my questions and suggested I talk again with Andrea Russo. I could ask her directly about what risks I was taking with the radiation therapy. She assured me that patients often had Brachy after chemo and that, by having postponed mine, I was not an outlier. I felt a little better and said that I would schedule another consult with Dr. Russo.

Then I took the elevator down one floor to Nisha. The ward was less busy that day, and she had time to chat. As she checked my infusion bags and hooked the tubes into my port, she reminded me that an increasing intensity of tiredness and other symptoms was normal for this fourth cycle. I should keep reminding myself that I was now more than halfway through it. I was doing well.

I reminded myself how lucky I was. My old high school classmate Audrey had called me "a lucky woman with cancer." My port had not caused any clotting or infections: my arms and hands were free to type. I was in a clean, bright, attractive ward, this time by an enormous picture window overlooking Boston. I had access to world experts and outrageous perks. I had as many Dixie cups of ice cream as I wanted to eat, and 20 minutes of acupuncture and massage with Michael, with whom I could discuss theater. What else could I want?

I could want not to have cancer, I thought. That was useless, I noted. It could have been so much worse. It could *be* so much worse. I could be in pain. I could be nauseous.

My bones could feel as though they were burning. How could I claim to be suffering? That was not a word in my vocabulary. My survivor parents rarely used it. It seemed not part of my culture. There were so many cultural dynamics in this cancer universe, I thought. Professional and religious community belief systems as much as gender and interpersonal chemistry.

Patrick picked me up and I was pink-cheeked as usual but considerably more subdued. When we got home, I noticed that I was walking more slowly. When I took my bath, I noticed that it had become harder for me to pull myself out of the tub, even with the steel handicapped bar that my son had installed. Patrick had begun hovering in the bathroom again after stopping for a time, ostensibly holding my bathrobe ready, but really – I knew – because he was so afraid that I would slip and fall.

I fell the next day. In my left hand was a glass with milkshake poured to the brim; in my right a glass of orange Gatorade and my iPhone. Obviously, I was not holding onto the railing – why would I do that, my muddled brain must have figured, I'm going *up* – not down. I have no idea why I stumbled but as I did, I watched myself go into slow motion. I was able to set down the glasses on an upper stair and watch them tip as I sank to my knees and slid, hoping that the glasses wouldn't break. The thick pink and thin orange liquids trickled down the staircase in two small rivulets. I wasn't badly bruised. But I had made a thud and Patrick came running. Now, in addition to monitoring my pills, hydration, temperature, blood pressure and blood oxidation, he began following me whenever I moved from one place to another. Several times a day, he'd ask, "Are you hiding anything from me?"

I knew that the thud of my fall had brought back the morning of my strokes, of which I had only a vague memory. I knew that he, on the other hand, still retained a traumatic memory of that day. But I got angry with his hovering and furious that he was adding to my burdens with his anxiety. “You want to know if I’m hiding anything?” I wanted to shout. “I’m hiding all the things I feel that will alarm you. I’m hiding that I can’t think straight. I’m hiding that I have to hold on to things in order to walk. I’m hiding that I feel poisoned and will get poisoned more.” Then I gave him a hug and asked him to please try to stop asking me questions.

September 29, 2020

Chemo Four, Day Five. A Tuesday. The weekdays and weekends had melded into one featureless loop. It was getting hard to keep track even of what month it was; I just felt that time was rolling downhill. I had experienced no steroid high this cycle – just wipeout. I had a headache and the margins of my vision shimmered in an ominous way. My joints and teeth ached. I felt off balance. My fingers and toes felt numb. I had no appetite, no energy. My brain felt clogged by sludge. I could do nothing but lie in my chaise and watch chipmunks and squirrels.

Was this the manifestation of what Nisha called, “cumulative fatigue?” Or was this an emergency? Patrick and I had instruments to measure other symptoms: a thermometer for fever, a blood pressure machine and oximeter for other vital signs. We had no way to measure blood count. Should I call the hotline?

Had anyone ever died of chemotherapy? I wanted to ask. My son Daniel was sure his friend’s mother had died of chemo and, much to my dismay, had told me so before I started. I would have googled "death from chemo," but I didn't even have the energy for that. Instead, feeling like a wimp, I once again called the 24/7 hotline. To my shock, AK herself picked up. She hadn't told me that in addition to performing surgeries, evaluating and counseling patients, teaching, and flying off to refugee camps, she regularly worked the emergency line. I was appalled to have reached her but so desperate that I asked, "How do I know I'm not dying?"

There was no way of assessing my exhaustion, I told her apologetically. Nothing to measure it, no baseline comparison. I couldn't even remember how I had slept that night. My surgeon's voice was soothing. AK said that in all her years of practice she knew no one who had died of chemo, that these low blood count days were very scary, and that people typically became anemic. She didn't think I was dying even though I felt as though I were, but that she would put in an order for blood tests and I should drive to the MGH near my home. Though I was not running a temp and my most recent labs showed no sign of one, I might have a urinary tract infection.

Why would she think that I had a UTI? And why was she so calm? It was hard to believe that my surgeon found my description of my physical state unalarming, the effect of cumulative chemotherapy. This was, apparently, par for the course: what happened when you slowly poisoned the entire body in order to eliminate the cancerous parts. It happened to all chemo patients – I wasn't an outlier. I tried to focus on the news: one million Covid deaths worldwide; widespread anxiety about the upcoming American presidential election; support for Black Lives Matter plunging from 54% to 19%. My friends were outraged and so was I but I had no breath to talk about it. I had spent the year writing political postcards to people all over the country with my Lexington group; now I had finally gotten too tired to even meet with them by Zoom.

Patrick drove me to have my blood drawn. He pushed me to keep drinking fluids and walk. I forced myself to walk the dog with him but moved so slowly that both of us became alarmed. At first, nothing improved. Then tests showed that I *did* have a slight urinary tract infection. AK prescribed antibiotics but they made my digestion worse. I stopped writing in my journals and stopped taking photos of my garden. The crisp air that usually elated me evoked only tepid pleasure. I was grateful for the fall foliage and for the fact that Patrick and I and both our sons – one in Michigan, one in Montreal – had managed to stay safe from Covid. But I lost interest in what people I loved were doing. I felt little about the imminent birth of my second grandchild. I recognized that these were symptoms of depression, items on that long list that had so annoyed me when I first started chemo. I knew that the hospital offered counseling services. But I was a veteran of psychotherapy and the thought of talking to a new therapist did not appeal. I continued to listen to music, to watch *The Crown,* to do my Italian homework every day. It became a major achievement for me to fill a blank in a sentence with the correct form of an Italian verb.

October 12, 2020

Finally, after two weeks, I felt better. I remembered Nisha explaining to me more than once that the infusion schedule included a week of recovery – in preparation for the next cycle. The weather was cooperating: it continued dry and warm, making it possible for me to continue to convalesce and entertain visitors outside. I was able to muster up some interest in news reports of President Trump's own bout of Covid. I managed to watch the Altman movie assigned by our film professor and not to miss a single Italian class. I started writing in my journals again. I was even able to bluff my way through a television interview for which I pulled a cloche over my bald head, passing for a religious woman wearing a head covering. Slowly, I returned to what I recognized as my usual self.

October 16, 2020

Chemo Five began well. The hospital had returned to a period of normal functioning. From the ninth floor, I photographed cars on the roof of the once-empty garage and, though carefully distanced, there were many patients in the waiting room. As she flushed out my port, Katie and I discussed President Trump's Covid treatment. The President was taking dexamethasone, the same steroid that I was taking, but Katie was sure it was a much larger dose. "He was all jacked up – 75 tweets in a matter of two hours." I jotted down her words. "They must have given him a lot." I thought about a writerly preoccupation: point of view. It interested me, every three weeks, to hear the medical staff's points of view on what was going on in our country.

My vitals and blood draws were normal. My infusion went without a hitch with Nisha giving me her own take on Trump, and acupuncturist Michael comparing making a living in playwriting and alternative medicine. After Patrick drove home, we had dinner and a long walk in the woods. *Seems stronger than last cycle*, Patrick wrote in his calendar. I felt so much better that I wrote an update to my email list.

Hello Everybody!

Five chemotherapy treatments down, one more to go and since I won't taper off the dexamethasone until tomorrow, I still have the energy to write an update. It's been a very long ride – but so many friends and family and neighbors came through!! That support has been invaluable...

Our mood is good. We finally feel we have run the gamut of side effects – not much more that can happen. I've learned that I cannot multi-task on chemo and Patrick is finally getting more comfortable with the ups and downs and is not as anxious this time.

And we are very excited about our second grandchild expected this month in Montreal.

That's the scoop for today. Be well, carpe diem, and please keep the emails and messages coming. I find them really helpful!!

<u>October 18, 2020</u>

Those steroids President Trump and I were taking were doing their job. I felt a little manic and finally wrote to radiation oncologist Andrea Russo that I was ready to reconsider Brachytherapy. But I requested some research studies.

I wrote, *I would like to read about:*

1) history and outcome of brachyiotherapy [sic] for endometrial cancer

2) What are survival outcomes per 100 patients (a high school classmate who had breast cancer, told me to ask)

3) when and why was chemotherapy added to radiation and what are comparative results of chemo only and radiation only?

4) does MGH have comparative studies of Brachy with and without chemo?

Thank you for scheduling me and answering whatever questions are not available in research studies.

Helen

<u>October 20, 2020</u>

Cycle Five, Day Five. Flattened again. I was unable to read anything. I felt so destroyed that I had little reaction to the news that my first granddaughter had just been born. Mother and daughter were doing well in Montreal though Covid was now wreaking havoc in Quebec. Great, I thought. That's over.

Despite the best efforts of the authors of *Chemotherapy and You* to prepare the patient for every eventuality, the prep depended on the patient not only reading it, but retaining and then remembering it. Each successive cycle introduced scary new symptoms that I found hard to describe. Every part of my body felt poisoned. The breakdown of my cognitive functions included memory, aphasia, inability to formulate or answer questions. I stopped wanting to listen to music or to read or write or even talk. All this while trying to keep calm *and* keep Patrick calm. He had vivid recall of my strokes and he was always ready to call 911.

Although I was spared nausea, I found the unpredictability of other symptoms terrifying, especially since they resembled what I read about Covid symptoms. I retained my sense of smell and taste. But I felt dizzy, breathless, achy, and was assailed by a stupefying mix of constipation, diarrhea, and acid reflux. The neuropathy in my fingers and toes now included occasional shooting pains in my heel, and a numbness creeping to my ankles. I had sudden toothaches and mouth sores that came and went. Chemo-fog had enveloped my brain with the density and all-pervasiveness of a real San Francisco Bay fog.

I forced myself to attend my 6 pm Italian class. My teacher and four classmates had witnessed my progress through surgery and chemo on their computer screens. Every Tuesday they saw me through various stages of hair and baldness. I felt comfortable with them and that Tuesday, thought that I could sit back, say nothing, and just listen. But we were doing gerunds and one of the students couldn't get it and kept mangling the verbs. Trying to follow the dialogue between her and our teacher became torture. I stopped being able to understand words, heard only garbled, meaningless sounds. That was so terrifying that I pressed, "Leave meeting." Fortunately Patrick was busy and didn't notice that class ended early. He served dinner and, afterwards, gripping the bannister, I dragged myself upstairs for a bath.

The bathtub was my refuge, the only place I still felt somewhat myself. It was a deep, six-foot tub surrounded by dark green tiles that I had chosen for their forest-like, soothing quality. For half an hour or so I soaked in the warm water, trying to process what had just happened. I was unable to. As I see it in retrospect, in addition to all its other powers, chemo can cause the equivalent of a severe learning disability. Though I've known several people with learning disabilities, I had never experienced one myself. My brain had almost always been able to provide optimal conditions to focus. Until it couldn't.

Patrick had lately decided not to monitor my entire ritual of washing, but nonetheless kept coming into the bathroom to make sure I hadn't drowned. I waved him away until he insisted it was time I got out. I grasped the metal bar and the side of the tub and tried to stand up. I couldn't. I didn't get upset. I thought it was funny: naked, tall, slippery, bald cancer patient trapped in tub, with tall strong clothed husband unable to pull her out. Patrick didn't find it funny at all. He instructed me to do this and that with my arms and legs. Nothing worked. Finally, with one of my legs hanging out over the bathmat, he hauled the rest of me out. I sat on the edge of the tub. Then I keeled over.

That wasn't funny. I had to concentrate hard on keeping myself from slipping to the floor. I don't remember ever feeling that weak before. No breath. No strength. No nothing except consciousness of trying to sit upright on the edge of the tub, staying still and trying to breathe. After a while, Patrick hauled me to my feet and led me to bed. Only months later did he tell me that the bathtub episode was right up there in scariness with the strokes. When he lifted me, it felt as though he was carrying dead weight – a corpse.

Later that night Patrick would write in his calendar the far less dramatic note, *8:45 pm when getting out of bathtub nearly falls, cannot sit up straight*. I fell fast asleep and, the next morning, was able to get out of bed and down the stairs on my own steam. But I was deeply frightened. I thought that I had never been so close to dying.

October 21, 2020

Cycle Five, Day Six. I had been able to secure an appointment with my acupuncturist Maribeth Kaptchuk. Patrick drove me into Cambridge, to the house around the corner from where we once lived. My concentration was shot, my reflexes were slowed, and he thought that I could keel over again at any moment. He had himself gone for a few sessions of acupuncture with our former neighbor but hated being pricked with a succession of fine needles. However, since AK had recommended acupuncture – to help detoxify the body after chemo, boost the immune system, and accelerate the healing process – he was putting his doubts and fears of virus contagion on hold, and working in the car while I had treatment.

Maribeth had suspended her practice when Covid numbers surged in Massachusetts but was seeing a few patients in her garden, under a tent that protected her equipment, the patient and herself from both sun and rain. She wore an N-95 mask covered by a face shield and homemade PPE. I wore a hospital mask and loose but warm clothing and lay down on the table. Her garden was stunning in all seasons and shielded from the street by a high wooden fence.

Maribeth practices Five-Element Acupuncture, a tradition that works with the life energy Chinese medicine calls *Qi.* I did not *enjoy* being needled, but in the 20 years I had gone for acupuncture whenever I felt depleted, it had always worked to both energize and relax me. I was fascinated by the theory: an organizing network of meridians along which *Qi* travels, that corresponds to specific organs like the heart or liver. I was amazed that I could track the movement of *Qi* in my body – like the illuminated route displays of the old Paris Metro – or feel an organ relax when *Qi* was released. The writer in me was also tickled by the evocative Chinese names of acupuncture points along the meridians, such as the Gate of Hope and the Palace of Weariness.

I also trusted Maribeth. Like AK, she was a woman of my time and place, with whom I could talk in cultural shorthand. Her garden was a healing place. It was late October, drizzling, almost the last week to be able to have this treatment outside. I desperately wanted to get back to my old self.

October 25, 2020

Cycle Five, Day Ten. My mind had cleared enough to think some. For one of her bouts of cancer, I remembered, my next-door neighbor Joelle had only five of her six scheduled cycles of chemo. My friend Rochelle's mother had stopped her chemo midway, when it became too difficult for her, and then lived for more than a decade. This was anecdotal rather than scientific evidence but it was enough to tip me over the edge and tell Patrick I, too, had reached the end of the line with chemo. I wanted to stop. Patrick, ever respectful of medical protocol, insisted that this was something that required discussion with AK; it could not be unilateral. I wrote her that day:

Dear AK:

This was an extremely difficult chemo cycle for me. I had and continue to have neuropathy in the feet and hands. My cognitive dysfunction was so bad that I had to leave my

Italian class because I could not follow it. I also had low blood pressure and breathlessness on days 4, 5, 6 to the point of not being able to stand up and went to Betsy Kaptchuk for acupuncture. It helped but I am very concerned about the neuropathy becoming permanent.

According to our notes, you explained to us that chemo significantly reduces the 20% risk of recurrence of serous cancer, but we can't seem to find to what extent. Do you have actual survival rate numbers? I am also wondering if you have statistics on patients who leave chemo before six cycles are up. Does completing six cycles make a major difference?

Dr. Russo sent me six papers to read but none of them mentions chemotherapy!! They all compare external radiation with Brachytherapy, as though chemo does not exist. For all these reasons, now that we have a better sense of what questions to ask, we would like to have a Zoom consult with you. How worried should I be about the cumulative effects of chemo? Should I get second opinion about continuing chemo and adding on brachytherapy? Could you recommend someone? Or do you think I am overreacting and everything I'm experiencing is just par for the chemo course?

Best,

Helen

I also wrote to Dr. Russo.

Dear Dr. Russo:

We have read the articles but they do not answer the question:

why do I need radiation therapy at all after surgery and chemo?

why is there no mention of chemo in any of the papers you sent me?

Are there any studies comparing outcomes that involve chemo with radiation? Chemo without radiation?

What are the benefits of radiation for someone with Stage 1A serous cancer who has had chemo?

Thanks,

Helen

<u>October 26, 2020</u>

Cycle Five, Day Eleven. Once again, things moved very quickly. Much to my amazement, AK called me and said I could stop chemo. That was a jolt. No problem! Done! Nothing to discuss! I had made a decision, taken control! I was totally relieved but Patrick, of course, worried if five cycles were really enough, why had I been prescribed six?

I thought about that too, but with anger rather than anxiety. Why put anyone through the torture of another cycle of chemo if you weren't absolutely sure it was essential? My ER doc classmate Audrey replied: *They push for 6 if tolerable. In medicine, it is always better to say we're doing 6 and settle for 5, than we are doing 5, and oh by the way, maybe we should do 6. It is a psychological win.*

But I had no brain space for what was now behind me. I was focused on Brachy.

Dr. Russo wrote:

If you are looking for a randomized trial of patients with serous stage I cancer who have received surgery and chemo and then randomized to radiation or no radiation, that does not exist…

There was no question of should you use radiation because use of radiation in early stage patients is considered standard of care. The question was 'do these patients need chemotherapy?' Please let my office know how you'd like to proceed or to set up an appt to discuss the literature.

How had both Patrick and I, in all our careful reading and consults, missed the fact that Brachy radiation was compulsory, or in medical jargon, "standard of care?" By then, I had learned to triage my questions. I could wait two days to hear what AK would tell us during our virtual consult. We celebrated The End of Chemo by driving to the beach, catching a late outdoor lunch on the empty terrace of our favorite seaside restaurant, eating clams and looking out at the waves. I walked slowly and didn't say very much but I felt as though a great weight had been lifted off my chest. Whatever lay ahead, I was relieved to have chemo behind me.

<u>October 28, 2020</u>

Day Thirteen, Patrick and I Zoomed with AK for 30 minutes, during which time I asked Patrick's (and my friends' and my classmates') list of questions: how comfortable was she with five rather than six cycles? Had any of her patients refused Brachy? How did survival rate per 100 compare between just chemotherapy alone to chemo and Brachytherapy for my kind of cancer? Would she mind if we asked for a second opinion?

AK was as calm and caring as usual. I worried that she would find us "difficult" but reminded myself that she had seen the gamut of patients and, given the givens, we were pretty easy. On second opinion, she gave us a name. On whether it made sense to stop chemo at Cycle Five when she had prescribed six, AK explained the need to balance efficacy of the treatment against possible permanent side effects. It was an art as much as a science. *The history is arbitrary*, read my notes. *Thirty years of data, trial and error and stats come from ovarian rather than endometrial cancer (serous behaves like ovarian cancer). In 1970s, women were getting two years. Then it was dialed back to one year. Then six months was going to be optimal. There is benefit in six cycles but not 100% of patients get there. In many situations, people have stopped at four.*

"Think of it as a convention rather than a rule," she told us.

With combination surgery, chemo and radiation, *recurrence is under 10%.*

If you take 100 women 50 will have it come back with no chemo. Don't have data on chemo with no radiation. When you don't eradicate all cancer cells they can come back very quickly so I should move ahead asap with Dr. Russo. Brachy will not affect me the way chemo did.

Once again, I could not compute the statistics but I trusted Patrick did.

Then she once again explained why Brachytherapy was "the standard of care."

Neither I nor Patrick had taken in or remembered reading that while chemo killed cancer cells everywhere in the body, it was less effective around stitches, particularly in the stitched-up area of the "vaginal cuff" – a kind of hem that now constituted the deep end of my vagina. Brachytherapy targeted those. That was important, especially since my cancer was serous, the most aggressive grade. Brachy was standard protocol and differed from abdominal radiation. It was local, limited, three short sessions. None of her hundreds of patients had ever reported side effects. Some even began in tandem with their first chemo cycle.

Now I felt stupid for not understanding this before and stupider for procrastinating. Having finally understood a key piece of information we had missed, we did not need a second opinion. I wrote to Dr. Russo and was given an appointment for November 10. I worried that I had procrastinated too long.

That day, we had another standoff with an unmasked dog walker. The Town of Lexington had instituted a mask mandate but few people observed it outside the town center, and especially not on the conservation lands that had narrow trails open to walkers and cyclists. Neighbors as well as strangers could walk their dogs, provided that they were either leashed or obeyed commands. Even in ordinary times, there were altercations with people insisting on their dog's "freedom to wander unleashed" or that their dog was "friendly." Typically, we called out to the owner when a dog came charging in our direction. I had even taken to using a whistle. Then, the owner would come running down the trail to argue rights and laws. Covid had considerably raised the ante. Even in liberal, highly-educated Lexington, many walkers saw no more reason to wear a mask than they did to leash a dog. That afternoon, Patrick – possibly more anxious than usual after our consult – had asked a young woman to please keep her distance and to wear a mask. She said she would report Patrick as a "stalker."

I did not need this kind of drama. The only places I was able to go were the hospital and the woods and streets in our neighborhood and that was becoming more and more difficult.

When we got back home, Patrick wrote to the Lexington Chief of Police so we would create a paper trail. I tried to calm down with breathing exercises. I had no energy for indignation. I was infinitely relieved to have no Cycle Six in my future but my body was still dealing with the cumulative effects of the previous five. I was bald all over, weak, unsteady, volatile. I aimed to strengthen myself physically and psychologically during the less than two weeks before the final stage of my cancer treatment.

October 30, 2020

Update #16

Big news is that, after starting what was to have been 6 cycles of chemotherapy on July 24, I asked if I could stop treatment at 5 cycles and my oncologist said YES.

My asking to stop chemo was a big deal. I didn't want to be difficult or noncompliant. But I felt that chemo was breaking me both physically and psychologically. I had managed five cycles. There are few guideposts to measure just how intolerable chemo is, how much worse it could be, how close you are to doing permanent damage to yourself. I found hard to even pinpoint and describe the many side effects. Although I was spared some of the worst such as nausea and mouth sores (just a couple of days), I had weakness and fatigue so bad that I could not stand up, and – most upsettingly – I couldn't think straight. I had an emergency number to call but no clear criteria re when to call. Sometimes there was a 15-minute wait. Sometimes the medical protocol (for chest pain for example) was to go to the ER – no discussion. I had been to the ER during Covid for strokes and didn't want to go back! I could measure the extent of my cognitive deficits most accurately every Tuesday during my Italian class. The worst one was after chemo 5, when everyone's words became gibberish and I found myself unable to follow the class. I saw myself as poor poisoned Russian Alexei Navalny, and had to sign out. I'm happy to report that this Tuesday (day 11 after chemo 5) I Zoomed back into Italian, and was able to follow. I'm hoping that acupuncture will make the neuropathy (in my toes and fingertips) eventually disappear. I am now focusing on detoxing my body and beginning brachytherapy on November 10. Everything should be done by my birthday (73) on November 27. After that, I will be on a three-month indefinite monitoring schedule by Dr. G. (blood tests, CT scans, physical exams) for the foreseeable future.

<u>November 3, 2020</u>

Election Day. We voted by mail. It was getting dark sooner and Halloween had been uneventful, but the weather remained warm. I could still put on a sweater, a hat, and maybe a blanket over my legs, and sit outside as though I was in an Alpine spa. It was now nearly six months since my diagnosis. My friends kept visiting – there weren't that many places you could get a good cappuccino and conversation, some joked – and so I listened to some friends worry about voting machines, Biden, Trump, violence. Part of me was anxious but part of me detached in a way I didn't recognize. I couldn't get up the energy to argue. Speaking still wiped me out after five minutes. A couple of days later, my writing partner Helen Fremont drove over for one of our regular sessions with homemade goodies and a piece of her new book to edit. My cognitive ability was back. I found that I could edit but was still unable to write. I couldn't even think about writing, I told my writing partner. I felt disaffected, as if I was removed by miles from everything. This was not new to Helen. Her wife has been a post-cancer patient for decades. "You've just been through a colossal bombing," she told me. "It's all-consuming, unpredictable. Add Covid. Add politics. Everyone else is at their wits' end, even without having to deal with cancer. It's too soon for you to write. You're not here. You will be again."

November 10, 2020

A highly unusual and very useful conversation with my brother Tommy, age 69, with whom I'd never before discussed our sexual organs. A few months earlier, he had undergone a Brachy procedure for prostate cancer, though his radiation was administered through radioactive "seeds" that had to be injected into his prostate rather than through a tampon. "You don't feel the radiation," he said. "The hard part is setting you up." He told me that two men came into the exam room before the procedure and he wondered why until the surgeon told them to hold him in place for the excruciating prep. Ugh.

Although I had already been measured for the tampon, I took an Ativan before we left. I walked down the stairs into the bowels of the building thinking of Dante's circles of hell. The chemotherapy ward was on the eighth floor, bright with windows, bustle, lots of people, and freezer cases of Dixie cups. Radiation was in the sub-basement: pea-green walls, no windows, no food, utter silence, like the morgue to which I went to identify my father's body after he died. Also, no matter how reassuring my brother Tommy had been, I was spooked by radiation. All those years of lead aprons at the dentist's, photographs of mushroom clouds, memories of The Twilight Zone.

I was now more or less resigned to Brachy – Tommy had gone through far worse, I told myself. No one would have to hold me down. It would not be painful. But the two-hour appointment did not proceed as planned. I was ushered into a small examination room and changed into a hospital gown. After a tech took my vital signs Dr. Russo, a petite complement to my medical team upstairs, asked about my emotional state and was very gentle in what was becoming a routine inspection of my vagina.

This time, however, that inspection yielded what my docs termed a "swerve."

Translated as "an unexpected development" in the form of a small, unfamiliar-looking "frond." I congratulated myself on having taken a sedative because Dr. Russo said she would need to clip off "the frond" and send it to be biopsied, before continuing treatment. She never uttered the words "malignant" or "benign" but I must have looked horrified because Dr. Russo reconsidered the situation and said: “well, I don’t think it’s anything serious and since you’re already here, we might as well do the measurements for the Brachytherapy so that if you come back next week, we’ll be all set to go.”

I understood by her “if” that if the growth turned out to be malignant, Brachytherapy was out and abdominal radiation was in. Dr. Russo measured my vagina for the Brachy tube, which I had read somewhere would feel like a Tampax made of lead. Even with a local anesthetic and lubricant, it did feel bulky and leaden. Measurements taken, I got dressed and made my way up to the street where Patrick was full of questions. The biopsy usually took two days. We each did our best to manage anxiety. The next day at 5 pm, Dr. Russo called with good news: the “frond” was benign.

The End? No. AK called, sounding apologetic but firm. “Out of an abundance of caution” could I come in for another biopsy? And would I mind having another PET scan? Not at all, I lied. Clearly she was worried. I didn’t mind having the scan but I dreaded the biopsy which, I knew would be very quick but painful. “80% of these are benign,” said AK before she cut. “20% are not.”

Results from that second biopsy would not come in until after the weekend. We binge-watched *The Queen’s Gambit,* walked in the woods, listened to the news as President Trump and his political surrogates refused to concede that he had lost the presidential election, tried to work. Finally, the mysterious “frond” was confirmed as benign.

November 12, 2020

Friends and neighbors knew only bits of what was going on. Some noticed that I had suddenly disappeared from view. I had no desire to tell anyone anything, no sense of obligation. I had no energy to help anyone else with their issues – whatever they were. Some people always feel this way. I never had. I noted that I had had to contract cancer in order to feel that I could put myself first. Remember this, I told myself. *You don't owe anyone anything*. I kept my focus narrow: eat, drink, walk, nap, breathe, sleep. Repeat.

Most people rolled with my erratic communications. They remembered what I had asked when I was diagnosed six months earlier: to hold their questions and advice, and if they wanted to make our lives easier, bring us food. So many of them had been through cancer that they knew the drill. But some didn't.

So it was that I found myself reading an email about a problem that had apparently been brewing for a month without my realizing it.

Dearest Helen,

I am so happy to watch your progress on FB. I have been going back and forth whether I should write to you. On one hand, I feel that we all have so much on our plates, why add more. But, on the other hand I have lost an important friendship because hurt feelings were not addressed in a timely manner.

It all started when we were scheduled to go over to your place with soup in hand. Then it was canceled last minute without explanation. I think what hurt my feelings was that you didn't give an explanation as to why. You didn't have to, but it would have been nicer. You might think it was not such a big deal, but for some reason it stung me. I was also willing to move on, because I knew how hard things were for you. It is also hard for me to acknowledge this, because you might think that it is so trivial...

She had noticed that I posted photos of other friends who had brought meals to us but none of herself and her husband, who had done so as well. He didn't know she was writing to me and I should not tell him. And so on.

At another time, I might have responded. I answer almost every email I receive. But I had no gas in my empathy tank. Instead, I had rage: could she not imagine what was going on with me? And she was a therapist! I let her email sit.

<u>November 14, 2020</u>

My friend who has been living with leukemia for 15 years had told me not to read anything about future problems until necessary. Now that I had my Brachy date, I decided it was time. I consulted the National Cancer Society website to learn the specifics of what a sassy friend called my "personal Chernobyl."

A source of radiation (a radioactive material) is put into a cylinder (called an applicator) and the cylinder is put into the vagina. (It feels a lot like a snug tampon.) The size of the cylinder and how much radiation is in it depend on each case. The upper part of the vagina, closest to the uterus, is always treated. With brachytherapy, the radiation mainly affects the area of the vagina in contact with the cylinder. Nearby structures like the bladder and rectum get less radiation exposure.

Treatment time is less than 20 minutes for 3 sessions. Common side effects of radiation therapy include tiredness, upset stomach, loose stools, and severe fatigue, which may not start until about 2 weeks after treatment begins. Diarrhea, nausea and vomiting may occur, but can be treated with medicine. These side effects tend to be worse when chemotherapy is given with radiation and are more common with external radiation.

I was glad I had waited till chemo was over.

Radiation can irritate the bladder, resulting in radiation cystitis, with discomfort, blood in the urine, and an urge to urinate often... Radiation can also irritate the vagina, called radiation vaginitis. Radiation can also lead to low blood counts, causing anemia.

Those were the possible short-term effects.

Long-term effects included vaginal dryness and scar tissue in the vagina, making the vagina shorter or more narrow. *A woman can help prevent this problem by having sex 3 to 4 times a week or by using a vaginal dilator. Vaginal dryness and pain with sex can be long-term side effects of radiation.*

Notwithstanding all this, once I had made the U-turn to Brachy, I stood by it. It was "standard of care." It wasn't Hiroshima. Tommy had done it. I was his older sister by three and a half years. I could do it too.

<u>November 17, 2020</u>

Dr. Russo's notes on my first treatment include:

Patient's identity was confirmed.

The patient was brought into the CT simulator where she was placed supine with knees bent. A cylinder was constructed and covered with a condom. It was coated with lubrication and inserted. The brachytherapy board was attached for immobilization. CT scan confirmed the appropriate depth of cylinder placement. A physics consult was requested. A graphic plan was generated and complex computer-optimized dosimetry performed. There were no complications.

The patient was brought to the HDR room. The cylinder size was confirmed, coated with lubrication and inserted to the vaginal apex. The brachytherapy board was attached for immobilization. The cylinder was connected to channel 1 of the Nucletron MicroSelectron High-Dose-Rate brachytherapy apparatus via the transfer tube. The attending physician reviewed the dosimetry, treatment plan, channel assignments and CT scan prior to the administration of radiation. All safety checks were performed including room and patient radiation survey. Radiation was delivered to the vagina with high-dose-rate Iridium 192 in 5-mm steps. The radiation oncologist and physicist were in the immediate vicinity at all times while HDR brachytherapy was administered. The functioning of equipment and the patient were continuously monitored by video and audio observation.

Following treatment, the room and patient were surveyed and were negative for radioactivity. The brachytherapy transfer tube and the applicator were then removed, and the patient was escorted out of the HDR room.

There were no complications.

<u>November 20, 2020</u>

My version:

On November 17, I had my first Brachy session in the subterranean exam room. The zapper looks like a Star Wars robot, maybe four feet tall and attached to a tube that attaches to the cylinder inside the vagina. You lie on your back, feet in stirrups, alone. You can choose your music and I asked for country western. They had problems with the machine and, after four lugubrious country western songs, I started thinking they had forgotten me. After 18 minutes, they came back. Thursday's session was even longer because the radioactive material requires that a physicist be present and they couldn't locate one of the two physicists on call. So once again I was left alone in the room with the robot. But radiation itself was no big deal. No sensation and no side effects so far at all.

This morning, at 7, we drove to Newton-Wellesley to have the PET scan that both oncological docs wanted. I had fasted; Patrick worked in the car while I went in at 8 am. At 8:30, a nurse apologized for the delay. The scan camera had broken down, the technicians had been called, but she couldn't say how long it would take to fix. Would I like to wait or reschedule? I didn't bother to consult Patrick, and asked: could I have it done at MGH downtown? She called her boss: they set it up, and scribbled my blood sugar results, the location of the lab and the name Steve, who would be waiting for me, on a scrap of paper.

They also gave me two containers of chalky "barium sulfate suspension" with straws. My husband should drive slowly: I should sip strategically en route and aim to empty the second container about five minutes before I had my PET. Patrick drove masterfully. I hopped out, sanitized my hands, took a new mask, and looked for the lab. There were two. At the first, the receptionist said there were two Steves. I called the phone number on my scrap of paper and was sent to the second lab. There were patients on gurneys and so busy they had no place to put me. The bustle put me in a much better mood than I had been in the basement, alone, being zapped. I got my PET scan and lots of attention. No one understood why I was so happy.

When Brachy was completed, Dr. Russo gave me a diploma for graduating.

<u>November 24, 2020</u>

My post-Brachy consult was next and focused directly on vaginal care. Mass General is as woke as it is well-endowed: along with acupuncture, nutrition, music therapy and massage, it maintained a Sexual Health Clinic, complete with private consults, workshops, support groups and online materials. Every member of the medical staff had offered me opportunities to talk about sex throughout my cancer treatment. Even before I had surgery AK had told me that, once my stitches had dissolved, I was good to go. Now, Nurse Practitioner Yoshie Sawin's job was to explain the mechanics.

Although I had grown accustomed to discussing my vagina, I was uncomfortable discussing my sexual life with a stranger. I had already read online that I was at high risk for vaginal stenosis, the shrinking and scarring that resulted from Brachy. *A woman can help prevent this problem by having sex 3 to 4 times a week or by using a vaginal dilator, a tube-shaped device that is inserted into the vagina. It is used to gently stretch it. This will allow your doctor to do pelvic exams. It is also important if you wish to be sexually active. Using a dilator is not the same as masturbation.*

I wondered who had written that and whether that was an attempt to disarm social conservatives. The daily news was filled with culture war issues.

Even my personal drama couldn't eclipse my worry about President Trump's continued refusal to concede that he had lost the 2020 election.

How do I use a vaginal dilator?

• *Find a place where you will be comfortable and able to relax.*

• *Choose a comfortable position.*

• *Before inserting the vaginal dilator, apply a water-based lubricant on the dilator and opening of the vagina.*

• *Gently insert the dilator only as far as it is comfortable. Gently move it forward and backward.*

• *Use your dilator for at least one minute.*

• *To remove your dilator, rotate it clockwise or counterclockwise, while gently removing it.*

How often should I use a vaginal dilator?

Use your vaginal dilator at least three times per week for at least one minute to start. Then, you can work up to using it from 3-10 minutes or as instructed by your health care provider.

Yoshie handed me a plastic bag with a silicone penis the color of a traditional, now obsolete, "Flesh" crayon and, very clinically, began talking vaginas. I thought of playwright Eve Ensler and her *Vagina Monologues*. Yoshie's speech would have fit right into it. I behaved as I had at the play: I watched and listened, but this time I didn't laugh. Unlike the schedule of 3 times a week I had read about online, Yoshie suggested that I use the dilator every night at first.

I nodded and stuffed the package into my handbag. Growing up on the West Side of Manhattan in the 1950s, I was regularly spooked by flashers and men masturbating on my way home from school. As an adult, I had never used sex toys; I spent years in psychotherapy working through childhood memories of sexual molestation. I wondered about the wide range of women who underwent what I saw as dildo-counseling and pitied Yoshie. She had a thankless job. I tried to be polite but got out of the basement as fast as I could.

Had I had a heart-to-heart with Yoshie, I might have said that my routine of pills, hydration, naps, and exercise made having sex seem like an additional chore. Pleasure, at that point, meant calm, not excitement; enjoyment without exertion. AK had reminded me that long marriage, meds, and prolonged stress all dampened libido. There was another thing too: cancer during Covid had fused my partner and me. In normal times, we led fairly independent lives. Since cancer and Covid, we had been eating every meal together, going to every medical appointment together, double-checking my every pill and test. We had, from the start, been a handholding, monogamous couple for whom sex was only one of many threads in a multi-textured fabric of connection. On his side, Patrick was still having flashbacks to watching me being loaded into an ambulance when I had my strokes. When I asked him whether he missed sex, he replied, "Yes but I'm afraid I'll hurt you." We both seemed relieved to defer resuming sex. I wondered how our stage of life and temperaments affected this. We had been married for 35 years and menopause had come on gradually for me – over a couple of years. What was it like to be 35 and have it happen in one day? What would it be like to have a partner who needed and/or demanded sex?

Three or four evenings a week, after brushing my teeth, I used my dilator as prescribed, took my pills, drank my large glass of water, read a lightweight book, then tried to go to sleep. Despite adhering to optimal "sleep hygiene," six uninterrupted hours was an elusive goal. I was lucky if I got four or five. Most nights, I did a body scan meditation, tensing and then relaxing successive parts of my body: eyes, mouth, shoulders, hands, buttocks, thighs, calves, ankles. Neuropathy had numbed my toes. It was hard to differentiate between my big toe and my second toe: on both feet, they felt frozen solid, like one big ice cube.

Chemo had undeniably damaged the nerves in my toes. The timeline for improvement was long and the damage could turn out to be permanent. I was lucky that the neuropathy in my fingertips had come and gone. Medicine did not yet have a cure for the condition. Although I hadn't heard or read it anywhere, I discovered that my toes preferred a steady temperature. They did not like hot baths or cold floors and were happiest in thick socks, so I wore socks all the time. My toes felt weird, but I could move them back and forth. Most of my torso felt dead. Once the discharge from surgery had finally stopped, my vagina and vulva had become bone dry and dead to sensation.

I sometimes ran my fingers over my bald pubis. A classmate who had undergone chemo wrote me that she was fond of her pubic hair and missed it even more than the hair on her head. I didn't mind losing mine. It was like opening a time capsule and remembering the body I had before puberty. What I missed were my eyelashes. I had never realized how *useful* they were in keeping dust and many particles out of my eyes. Before I fell asleep, I envisaged scenes from the last trip Patrick and I had taken, to the jagged Dolomites, where we had seen thousands of sheep on the mountainsides. The pills did their work. I'd fall asleep.

<u>November 26, 2020</u>

Thanksgiving Day, my favorite holiday. It always fell around my birthday and, in addition to turkey, my memories were of presents and chocolate cake. When I was a child, we lived a block away from Central Park West where the Macy's Parade passed by. We'd spend the morning watching the enormous balloons and floats and come back to an apartment that smelled divine. My mother always made sweet Czech stuffing with almonds and raisins – a tradition I continued. This time, of course, there was no extended family. Six of its members had already had Covid and no one was traveling. We had Thanksgiving by Zoom and ordered dinner from a local restaurant. The flavors were unfamiliar but my appetite was back. I noticed that around that time both Patrick and I stopped tracking my symptoms in our respective calendars.

I also finished reviewing a book I had begun reading before my diagnosis six months earlier: a 600-page scholarly biography. I love reviewing good books, an activity that draws me deeply into a text and a community of writers and readers for whom books matter. Now, after the brain ravages of chemo, I took pleasure in the process of rereading the biography, and taking copious notes. It seemed to take me twice as long, but I managed to write a cogent review. *My brain is back*, I thought when friends commented on it. *It's just a little clunky*. And I take great pleasure in writing. Like so many writers, I find that it helps me understand what I think.

<u>December 4, 2020</u>

My son Daniel gave me an elegant set of knives for my birthday. Probably not the best choice for a person recovering from chemo. I was super-conscious of the newness and sharpness of the knife and unaware of any neuropathy in my hands. I tried to be extra careful but managed to slice into my thumb instead of into the zucchini I was cutting for dinner. It didn't hurt much but bled and I remembered I was taking a blood-thinner. It bled through one napkin, then two. I didn't want to go to the ER. I bound it up with paper towels and layers of cotton gauze and didn't take my blood-thinner that night. In the morning, the gauze was red and I called Dr. Bala who happened to be seeing patients in person that day. She was concerned but unalarmed, and I felt happy to be seeing her about a household accident – not cancer. Her assessment read:

has a clean 1/2 inch cut on her left thumb. Attributes to doing things while talking to husband rather than neuropathy. Did not want to go to the ER. She was worried as she is on apixaban. Hence, she did not take blood thinner last night and not this morning either due to concerns for bleeding.

- *On exam, noted no signs of infection.*
- *Clean cut is easier to heal.*
- *Will apply steri-strip to close the wound which also gives enough pressure to stop the bleeding. Will ask the nurse to give her some extra dressing to take home.*
- *Advised to focus on the task when performing activities like cutting with a sharp knife.*

Dr. Bala reminded me that I had just been through an extraordinary five months and I needed to be mindful of ordinary routines in order to avoid injury. It was not over yet. It would be a few more months until I was back to anything like my old self. I left feeling cared for and, as so many times that year, infinitely grateful to my team of doctors.

On the occasional warm day, I still enjoyed being outside – lying under blankets in my chaise like a convalescent in *The Magic Mountain.* The temperature still reached 60 at noon. Sometimes I tried to rake leaves or prune a bush but got so tired after 10 minutes that I had to sit down and rest. Though the trees were bare, the warm weather held almost until Christmas and friends kept visiting and drinking Patrick's lattes on our lawn. The number of people willing to sit and chat outside in their down jackets had dropped considerably however, and Patrick would not allow anyone inside our house. The global count of Covid deaths had reached 1.7 million by then. In Massachusetts, the number of cases was spiking after Thanksgiving family get-togethers and Patrick wasn't taking any chances with anyone – including our sons. We would have loved to hold our infant granddaughter in Montreal but the border was closed even if Patrick could have been persuaded to travel to Canada and we waved at her on Skype.

The only indoor spaces I entered were the hospital and my acupuncturist's office. It always energized me and provided a sympathetic witness who recorded my recovery. Maribeth's needling had managed to unfreeze my big toes from their neighbors: they no longer felt fused. And conversation was an important part of the treatment. We had known one another, our partners and children for some 20 years and could talk politics or books or indulge in the kind of casual conversation that had disappeared during the pandemic: what our partners and kids were doing, what mini-series we were watching. I was now taking great pride in driving myself to Cambridge and back solo.

Without naming names, Maribeth told me about the arcs of recovery some of her other cancer patients had followed. I was also culling useful tips from reading, including the late Gilda Radner's book about her ovarian cancer; Susan Gubar's *Reading and Writing Cancer: How Words Heal;* then Siddhartha Mukherjee's encyclopedic *The Emperor of All Maladies: A Biography of Cancer.* Each one of them was useful in its way, giving me new angles of insight into what I had experienced and not yet processed, and what I was experiencing now. Those insights felt like gifts and made me want to write my own account of treatment and recovery. When I told friends what I was thinking, they said it was a sure sign of health.

<u>January 6, 2021</u>

As we drove to my Brachy follow-up, we listened to reports on the radio of thousands of Trump supporters massing in Washington, D.C. two weeks before the inauguration of the new president. Everyone I knew was on edge, especially people whose families – like mine and Patrick's – had fled totalitarian countries for democratic ones, sensing the not so outlandish possibility of a coup. They were checking their phones for the latest news, cabin-feverish from pandemic seclusion, lonely, scared. I descended down to the Radiation basement, thinking of Dante and dungeons again. At least I was leaving politics behind. The grim realities of radiation trumped even Trump. Every time I went for an appointment down there, I wondered what combination of psychological mechanisms enabled staff to continue working there. It was like working on a nuclear submarine.

Helen is doing very well, Yoshie wrote in my chart. *Has used the dilator daily and also sexually active, will reduce dilator use to 2x/week. Aware intercourse can take the place of dilator as long as done on a regular basis.*

She will follow-up with Dr. AK Goodman in February and Dr. Russo in May. She is aware to call sooner with questions or concerns. All of her questions were answered to the best of my ability.

"Doing very well" and "sexually active" were pushing it. Patrick and I had tried having intercourse once or twice and had given up. He was still thinking about my stitches and radiation and worried about inadvertently injuring me. Both of us disliked following AK's recommendation of "lots of lube." We were, I think, feeling not sexual desire but a desire to be back to normal. We let it go for a while.

New England winter had finally begun for real. It was cold and, six months after starting chemo, my hair on my head was only about a quarter of an inch long. The good news was that everybody was wearing hats, so that mine no longer looked unusual. My energy level could reach about 75% on a good day. I had even given a Zoom talk at my local library book club about writing non-fiction. What was different and probably would always be different from pre-cancer was that I followed a rigid daily practice of medication and self-care.

I still couldn't get enough sleep, even with napping almost every day – something I had never done before cancer. I still couldn't hydrate enough to stop my legs and hands from cramping. I had vestiges of chemo-brain: faulty memory, word loss, problems with dates and numbers. Well-meaning friends told me that they were having similar issues, attributing them to age and/or Covid but I didn't buy it. I'd always had an excellent memory. I'd also always been an enthusiast, with very little ambivalence about any project I undertook.

Now I felt unenthusiastic and ambivalent about almost everything. That was a shock. Not like myself. I was expecting to have my pre-cancer stamina back, but still tiring after an hour's conversation. My roller coaster ride of crises, however, was beginning to even out: no more unexpected dips or swerves or fronds. A slow but steady trek towards health.

Emotionally, however, I had just begun to process cancer.

February 5, 2021

Patrick got teary as he drove me to my appointment with AK. It was my first post-treatment check-up and he was anxious, as were some of my friends. I wasn't thinking about whether my cancer was gone or not. I was thinking about how many Covid patients were in the building, how many staffers had caught the virus, how my team was holding up, how many had been vaccinated and when I'd be able to get my shot.

The drill was still the same as it had been for months: no significant others, hand sanitizer, new mask. Patrick found parking and opened his laptop to work. Since my diagnosis, he had acquired and digitized twenty eBooks.

Now, as he settled in with Leon Blum's memoir of the Dreyfus Affair, I took the elevator up and checked in. In normal times medical visits often seemed like an annoyance; after eleven months of Covid, visiting the large cast of characters on the ninth floor was a welcome social event. At the reception desk, I was offered a choice of colorful hand-crocheted beanies made by a volunteer. I put on one with a rainbow pattern. My tech had been pregnant for much of my treatment; now I wished her an easy delivery as she took my vital signs and ushered me into AK's exam room. Then Katie came in to flush out my port and draw my blood.

By now, I hated my port. It was like an enormous plastic tick that I couldn't pull out. Winter sweaters usually disguised the bulge it formed but I was conscious of its weight under my skin for what seemed every single minute of the day. It had been an extraordinarily efficient way to deliver chemo and test blood. But now that chemo was over, I wondered when it would come out. Katie said nothing about that as she worked, so I raised the subject. I had read that ports needed flushing every six weeks to prevent infection and clots, I told her. My follow-ups were every three months. So shouldn't I have it removed?

"Up to you," said Katie. "Some people want it out; some people leave it in."

That was pure Katie, I thought. Clearly she herself had never had a port implant. The unspoken question, I supposed, was how soon will you have a recurrence of cancer and need it again? Once again I wished MGH, which seemed to have everything else, had a case manager. But maybe, I reflected, this was part of post-cancer care, encouraging the patient to start making her own medical decisions without the pressure of time. I asked Katie for the details of how it was removed. The *explant* – a new word for me – was very much like the implant, she said: a shot of lidocaine; an incision; they took it out; they stitched up the cut. "No big deal. You'll just have to consult your doctor about when to stop your blood-thinner."

Explant was mini-surgery but surgery nonetheless. Unlike my refusal to countenance radiation and my U-turn to accepting it, deciding whether to remove the port was more like a seesaw. One day yes; one day no. What if I had the explant and was obliged to implant again? On the other hand, I already had a blood-clotting problem, why would I add to it? Katie might think the decision was no big deal but, to me, it felt huge. I didn't think that stopping my blood-thinner for a couple of days would cause a stroke. But deciding what to do about my port felt major. Taking it out meant a vote of confidence in being cancer-free. Leaving it in meant a vote for cancer recurrence. But Katie wasn't a shrink and I didn't feel comfortable having this discussion with her.

AK didn't have the time for psychotherapy either. It was February and I noticed that our periodic consults had shortened considerably. She had been working throughout the pandemic with barely any time off, worn out by the pandemic and politics. I didn't want to burden her with my port anxieties. I was doing very well, I told her when she asked. Acupuncture seemed to be helping the neuropathy in my toes. I was taking the supplements she recommended. I needed fewer naps. My sleep and digestion weren't great but what else was new? Then AK lowered the examination table, inserted her speculum and checked out my vagina for spots or growths like the "frond" Dr. Russo had discovered before Brachy.

Nine months in, pelvic exams had become as routine as eye or dental exams for me. Spreading my legs with feet in stirrups, I made conversation with AK as she worked, telling me what she was seeing while she did. Many instruments had probed my insides while I was conscious, unconscious, or dissociated. Just as I had done while receiving my chemotherapy, I had refused to look, refused to take in what was happening. Maybe that explained my rage at having to now undertake the vaginal dilator regimen. That on top of all the other invasive routines, they wanted *me* to stick something into myself? But there was no point in burdening AK with all this. I had to do it or my vagina would shrivel up like a raisin and not only would I never be able to have sex again, but she wouldn't even be able to give me a proper exam. No point discussing it.

When I looked at AK's after-visit notes for that day, I read:

Feels great. Is planning to write a book about her experience

CT Chest Scheduled for 5/3/2021

CT Abdomen/Pelvis Scheduled for 5/3/2021

February 14, 2021

In fact, I was not feeling great that Valentine's Day. Patrick had not been raised celebrating it and whenever I complained, he said, "Every day is Valentine's Day with you." Apart from neuropathy in my toes, most of my side effects had disappeared or stabilized. But emotionally, I was unpredictable. Up. Down. Vivacious. Limp. Patrick was terrified that I would catch the virus and insisted on doing all our errands and shopping. Except for my medical appointments and weekly visits to my acupuncturist, I was under house arrest. The only place I drove was to my acupuncturist's office through a desolate Harvard Square. There were no students and it was too cold for anyone else to be outside for long. When I had the energy, I talked to friends on the telephone and read and wrote. I went on Zoom to tutor my Parisian niece; take my Italian class; take my film class; talk to friends. It was treacherous to walk on the icy streets or in the woods. I tried to exercise indoors and got irritated, especially with Patrick.

His 67th birthday was February 10. I pulled off a surprise Zoom party with cake, candles, both sons and grandson. I thought it a major accomplishment, but forgot that Patrick didn't celebrate his birthday more than any other holiday. After the Zoom, that and everything else about him enraged me. He had bought instant Tapioca instead of Tapioca pearls. He needed an aisle map of every supermarket. Whenever a thought crossed his mind, he needed to inform me immediately, no matter what I was doing, like a toddler. I knew that he had been in emergency mode since my strokes. I knew he was afraid I'd die and leave him alone. I understood PTSD. But in the moment, I didn't care.

The next day I woke up infinitely sad. We wound up slowly making love for the first time since my surgery. It wasn't anything like before cancer but at least it was a start.

February 17, 2021

Patrick drove me to the medical outpost where I had had the implant on July 20. After seven months of having a foreign body in my body, I was more than ready for the explant. But both of us were anxious. There would be no general anaesthetic and, as usual, I worried about the pain of the cut. Patrick worried, as usual, that the surgeon might be drunk. The risk of contagion was a given by now. I kissed him good-bye, put on a new mask, used the hand sanitizer, greeted the receptionist, changed into a hospital gown.

A female nurse settled me onto the gurney, draping a sheet discreetly over my body. For the first time, I had a duo of men: a male tech and a male doctor. This startled me. I had grown accustomed to being taken care of by women.

“Good temp, beautiful blood pressure,” boomed the tech, checking my chart. “There’s usually no complications. It’ll take longer to prep and drape than to take the thing out. First we clean the skin. Then we numb it up.”

Ryan instructed me to keep my hands beside my body, lowered my sheet to mid-breast, and scrubbed the top of my chest vigorously with an antibacterial solution. I closed my eyes, opening them only when I heard him greet the doctor. He was young, long-haired and looked like a hippie who had just rolled out of bed. I was glad Patrick couldn’t see him.

Dr. X said almost nothing. I closed my eyes again, felt the push of the needle injecting lidocaine into my chest, the pressure of a cut, then I heard the sounds of stitching. The tech had not lied. The explant took less than five minutes. The doctor left without a word. In the dressing room mirror I saw a large bandage above my right breast. I had done my research. I knew I would have:

Soreness

Possible bleeding

Minor discomfort at site

No baths for two weeks

No lifting or strenuous activity for a week

I was warned that the wound might appear healed in 2-4 weeks, but would take 2-3 months to be fully healed and that scarring was inevitable.

I didn't care. The tick was finally out. I didn't need to take a painkiller and I had no bleeding or infection. I celebrated by diving into a book I'd been asked to review. And I resumed (via Zoom) a book tour that had been canceled before it began.

In February of 2020 – exactly one year earlier – I had been preparing to travel for *Franci's War*, a Holocaust memoir written by my late mother. She had been a dressmaker in Prague who survived the concentration camps by pretending to be an electrician. It was being published in eight countries, starting with the U.S. and UK. Just before Covid broke out, I was being trained by a former BBC interviewer to hype the book to British readers. Readings had been scheduled in Boston, New York, Washington, D.C., London and Prague.

Everything had been canceled. But several of the venues had immediately switched to Zoom. I did my first Zoom reading on March 24. In May, cancer forced an interruption in the schedule. Now, a year later, I put on dangly earrings to offset the super-short hair that made me look like a punk rocker, and Zoomed with a book group in Israel. I had three more book talks scheduled in March. The long-distance Q and A was exhausting but it felt very good to be an author again – not a patient.

March 3, 2021

I got my first Covid shot a few days before Patrick: a Pfizer vaccine at MGH. Vaccine rollout in Massachusetts had been unexpectedly slow and disorganized, lagging behind other states. Governor Charlie Baker initially withheld vaccines from hospitals. Patrick, for his part, refused to trust any institution besides Mass General.

Baker's mistakes only added to the disgruntled mood. Cabin fever in New England always hit its apex in March, but this year people were going really crazy with isolation. The weather was dismal. The new president and vice-president were a solace to me but the political news was discouraging as was climate news and pandemic news. Yet everyone kept scanning the headlines on their phones. We subscribed to newspapers in the U.S., France, and Israel – too many. Friends were cracking under the strain of information overload or being cooped up with small children or adult children with disabilities whose daycare had been canceled. And some of my women friends were being diagnosed with cancer.

Just as I was coming out of the treatment tunnel, two emailed that they were entering it. Both of them had stage 3 endometrial cancer and both were MDs. The first asked if she could consult me as she went through treatment.

It is so surreal going through this experience during Covid, she wrote. *I was given an OR date but advised that it could very possibly be cancelled due to the pandemic. All I want right now is to start moving this process forward so I can get past it. I have closed my practice this week so I can focus on my recuperation from surgery, and treatment. I've been thinking of contacting you but always procrastinate. I think it may be because I've done better than I expected so far and I'm afraid I'll jinx myself if I say that. Lots of room for magical thinking in cancer land.*

I remembered AK telling me that gynecological cancer was the fastest growing cancer among women and that no one knew precisely why.

March 15, 2021

My acupuncturist Maribeth had moved into her HEPA-filtered office when the weather got cold, with her patients and herself wearing masks. Driving the six miles from Lexington to her Cambridge office – still the only driving I did by myself – became a highlight of my week and one of my only regular in-person social interactions.

Since *The Yellow Emperor's Classic of Internal Medicine* was written around 100 BCE the Chinese practice of acupuncture had spread to many countries. Some schools encourage conversation, some work in silence. Some practitioners needle for ten minutes, others an hour. Sometimes, as I lay on my back, my interaction with Maribeth reminded me of psychoanalysis. I noticed and said what came into my mind.

Cancer was a watershed: I had been sailing along taking life for granted and then suddenly had lost all the givens as well as all control. Now I was slowly trying to figure out my post-cancer world, sifting through what was essential and what was not, what people and activities I wanted to retain in my life, which friendships I might let go. Cancer had bonded me more deeply to some friends and cut loose others, including some decades-long relationships. For the first time in my life, I felt as though both my time and energy were limited. I felt a little stupid about this, I told Maribeth. As if I were discovering something that lots of other adults had long known. But the truth was I was feeling for the first time in my life that I couldn't carry as much as I had been carrying. Too much. I always knew that all relationships required investment but now I realized how much some had been draining me. I had over-invested. I felt that in my body. I wanted a rest. I wanted to put out less and take in more. I wanted to be taught Italian, or film or about acupuncture. I didn't want to put out in any way.

In five-element Chinese medicine, Maribeth said as she needled points along the liver, small intestine and heart meridians, the kind of sifting process I described was seen as the purview of the small intestine. Its function was to digest and sort pure from impure, separating what to keep from what to jettison.

As I had done for years in psychoanalysis, I listened carefully to my therapist and then to what came into my mind. My gut, in fact, had been a problem for most of my life. Some people developed headaches when they were stressed; I had always developed stomach aches. Chemo had only exacerbated what had been for me a life-long problem: I stuffed stress, not into my back or shoulders or head, but into my gut. As Maribeth needled the meridians, my digestive tract relaxed. It never failed to amaze me, this invisible yet clearly direct link between points on my arms or legs and my internal organs but it was powerful. *Qi* moved through my body in ways that I could easily track. Except in my toes, which though less frozen together, were still disappointingly numb.

Maribeth needled the spaces between my toes. My doctors and people who suffered from neuropathy told me I was very lucky not to have pain along with numbness. Toes, I was told, were at the very end of the longest nerves in the body. They ran from my spinal cord, down my very long legs to the end of my long feet. *Qi* never seemed to get to them, no matter what Maribeth did and I had heard that it took years after ending treatment to get anywhere near back to "normal." If ever. Some things ended. It was hard to accept but true.

I had just Skyped the evening before with a friend who knew that in her being. I might have grown up with Eva in Prague had my parents not fled Communism. She was a book editor, theater person, former dissident, wife, mother of three, grandmother of five, daughter of a concentration camp survivor like me.

We spoke Czech together and, maybe because I have to think and search for the right words more carefully when I speak my childhood language, I began to reflect more deeply on the passage I had been navigating.

Eva asked about my recovery and told me that she, too, had just had laparoscopic surgery. Not for cancer, but still a total hysterectomy – uterus, ovaries, etc – in a Prague hospital so packed with Covid patients that it had been difficult to get any nursing attention. She had been glad to get back home and back to work. She shared my take on our reproductive organs. "They've done their job," Eva said. We were both well over 60.

I had watched several of my friends, after hysterectomies, obsess over their continuing attractiveness, as well as death. Eva, who had always been strikingly beautiful, skipped over the issue of desirability and went straight to death. She said that if she had died, it would not have been a tragedy. She had lived a full life. I felt the same way. I remembered a poem that my late father often used to recite in Czech. I never knew what prompted it. Maybe the poet or the poem had figured in his life in a way that I, an ocean, a culture and an age removed, would not have understood anyway. The line he liked the best was, roughly translated, "Death isn't evil; it's just a difficult piece of life."

April 6, 2021

I returned to writing for a few hours every morning, as had been my practice before cancer. The publishing industry all over the world was struggling back to life and I still had correspondence and promotional obligations.

Doing ordinary things was thrilling. I drove to the supermarket for the first time in over a year. I could handle the interstate but the enormous parking lot filled with moving carts, cars, and pedestrians rattled me. My cognitive function, I noted, was still far from 100%. The supermarket seemed gigantic: the quantity of things packed high on both sides of the aisles and multiple choices of milks and yogurts and ice creams overwhelmed me. I'd forgotten how shoppers behaved, browsing at different speeds, stopping without warning, and what products were in which section. Patrick had ordered me to prepare a list, itemized by aisle, and move quickly – not linger but grab and get out as fast as I could. Instead, I found myself taking pleasure in looking at long unseen boxes and cans and bottles, ignoring the danger of being in a large indoor space with the exhalations of strangers. Buying groceries felt like a luxurious indulgence.

I took even more pleasure in being a student again, newly appreciative of the workings of my brain. In addition to my Italian and film classes, I joined one of the online book groups that had sprung up since the pandemic began. We spent six meetings on Israeli author Batya Gur's *Murder on the Kibbutz*, doing close textual analysis of the kind I hadn't done since college. Batya was a very special author for me. Uncertain of her talent in the highly patriarchal Israeli literary scene, Batya had only started writing her first novel at the age of 39 and, as her *New York Times* obit noted, was "almost single-handedly responsible for making the detective novel a flourishing genre in Israeli letters." She was born a few months before I was, a daughter of Holocaust survivors, a graduate of my university, an author steeped in psychology. And she had died at 57 of cancer.

April weather was iffy but even though I got winded after 20 minutes, I was able to poke around my garden. I felt grateful for those 20 minutes and grateful to fall onto my wooden bench and stare at the snowbells and croci and daffodils that had emerged from beneath the snow.

After the narrowing of my consciousness as well as capacities over the past year, I had become aware of how deeply I felt excitement, enjoyment, curiosity, losing myself in contemplation and following with interest developments in the lives of others. While I continued to be annoyed by Patrick's micro-management (it was taking him longer to adapt to my vastly improved state of being) I realized how essential he was to me. As a friend had confided about her late husband, "He was nuts about me and it was very healing."

With friends, I began to move slowly back toward my more characteristic supportive role. I listened attentively but noticed that I didn't pepper them with questions the way I had done before cancer. I had learned during my treatment that being questioned could feel like being interrogated and invaded and that people often didn't want to answer my questions. I still didn't want to see anyone who required an expenditure of energy. More than reflecting about death, I was reflecting on new ways of coming back to life.

April 23, 2021

My hair was growing back in. It looked and felt unrecognizable: same pepper-and-salt color but completely different texture. Chemo-curls. When I ran my hand through my hair I felt as though I was caressing Patrick. *Hair grows back differently for everyone,* one of my candid former classmates informed me. *My pubic hair came back less full but different, long and soft. I'm fond of it. Return of strength is more gradual. Even though I had just finished radiation, I felt pretty good after 6 months; I still tired more easily from long days but not from short walks. Took about a year until I was back at 90% and a year after herceptin for full recovery of energy. This was about 10 years ago: it might be a bit slower in our aged selves but there is a great deal of individual variation. Also, I have alas never been an energetic person.*

In the news, we heard that Covid was spiking dramatically in India, but in the U.S. where over 30 million cases had been reported, a kind of lull had set in. My son Daniel, who was 35, had his first jab of vaccine. He had been calling almost every night from Michigan, but now fell back into his more usual pattern. People we knew had settled into their Covid-time professional routines and no longer had as much free time. Although I had set up an outdoor visiting space and friends continued to come by, they no longer saw me as a patient and stopped delivering treats. I was very happy to be recovering well but noticed that I missed the attention. Apart from Patrick, only Kashu remained my devoted companion.

May 8, 2021

An unusually cold Mother's Day. Every year, our older son would send flowers. The morning before, our doorbell rang. I peered through the window and saw a man standing on the steps, his face obscured by a wide-brimmed hat.

"Flowers!" he mumbled. I didn't open the door.

"Are you wearing a mask?" I asked, before Patrick rushed over shouting. "Are you wearing a mask?"

"Yes," the deliveryman said. The man's hat was hiding most of his forehead and the mask covered his nose and mouth. Patrick asked him to leave the flowers on the bench, but the man refused, saying he needed a signature.

Patrick opened the door part way and reached for the paper. The deliveryman handed him a bouquet, asking, "Don't you recognize me?" It was our older son Daniel. Fully vaxxed. Looking great. We stared in amazement and hugged him. We hadn't seen each other in person in over a year.

I had sailed blithely through my scheduled CT scan a few days earlier. If I was going to have scans and exams every few months for the next five years, I had decided there was no point wasting energy on worrying. I was more concerned about other people I knew who had unexpected medical issues that week.

Patrick, of course, was anxious about my results. He kept asking if I had heard from AK, but I received no notification about the scan. That too, it seemed, had devolved to being the patient's responsibility. When it finally occurred to me to check my online medical record and read through the report, I made out the key phrase: *No abdominopelvic metastases*.

We celebrated with Daniel.

May 27, 2021

One year after my diagnosis of cancer, I had a six-month follow-up with radiation oncologist Dr. Russo. I still got the creeps in the MGH oncology clinic but assumed that my treatment had killed off the cancer. Dr. Russo noted:

Ms. Epstein was last seen in this clinic by Yoshie Sawin on 1/6/2021.

Since that time, she had her port explanted and has continued to be followed by Dr. Balasubramaniam, and Dr. Goodman. She was noted to have most likely chemotherapy-induced peripheral neuropathy that is expected to slowly improve over time.

Today, Ms. Epstein reports feeling generally well though notes that she has no libido. She has not experienced any vaginal bleeding or discomfort. She continues to use the dilator weekly.

Dr. Russo said I'd be able to stop using my dilator in the fall and that, unfortunately – because of my type of cancer – I could not prod my libido with hormone replacement therapy. Once again, she mentioned the hospital's Sexual Health Clinic. Once again, I didn't call.

June 15, 2021

In the news today:

CNN's chief international anchor Christiane Amanpour told viewers Monday that she has been diagnosed with ovarian cancer.

Amanpour was 63 years old. I had long admired her directness in reporting the news. Now she applied the directness to her illness:

I'm now undergoing several months of chemotherapy for the very best possible long-term prognosis, and I'm confident, Amanpour said. *From her home base in London, Amanpour said she wanted to "urge women to educate themselves on this disease; to get all the regular screenings and scans that you can; to always listen to your bodies; and of course to ensure that your legitimate medical concerns are not dismissed or diminished."*

August 18, 2021

Patrick drove me into Boston for my third follow-up. The skin on my chest where the port had been was smooth now and Katie drew my blood from my arm. AK came in, wearing her pointy cowboy boots. In this second summer of the pandemic, she still looked like she badly needed a vacation but was as calm and receptive as always. When she asked how I was feeling, I told her about Christiane Amanpour. When she asked about my physical state of being, I told her that things were pretty good except for my toes. She repeated what I knew, that the last small stretch of recovery took a very long time.

I don't know what she read in my face – we were still wearing masks and it was hard to read anything – but she told me about a friend of hers, who had had lymphoma. Years later, she knew that she was finally going to make it when she stopped trying to memorize all the things in her environment. "Her return to taking things for granted was such a gift," AK said, "I wish that for you."

Then she reminded me of the medical protocol for the next five years.

Year One: Physical Exams (abdominal check, pelvic exam) and labs every 3 months. Mammogram yearly.

Year Two: Exams and labs every 4 months.

Year Three, Four and Five: Exams and labs every 6 months.

Other Follow-up: Yearly chest and abdomen/pelvic CT scans unless there is a new symptom or concern.

I wrote it all down in my notebook. We hugged, even though we were still wearing masks.

"Watch out for blood in the vagina," she said. "See you in three months."

Acknowledgments

It takes a village to heal a cancer patient.

First, I salute and thank my outstanding and extraordinarily kind team of medical professionals: in chronological order Dr. Devasena Balasubramaniam, Dr. Uchechi Amy Wosu, Evelyn Durand, Dr. AnneKathryn (AK) Goodman, Kathleen (Katie) E. Megan, Maria Avila-Wallace, Dr. Andrea Russo, Yoshi Sawin, Nisha Wali, Dr. Aneesh Singhal, Dr. Johanna Helenius, acupuncturists Maribeth Kaptchuk and Michael Kearny and all the welcoming technicians, receptionists, and volunteers whose names I never got to know.

Second, I thank my family, especially my brothers Tommy and David Epstein, my sisters-in-law Susan Zales and Dawn Cavrell, my sons Daniel and Sam Mehr, and my daughter-in-law Alia Martin for being there in crucial ways.

Third, I thank my friends and neighbors who nourished me: above all next door neighbor Joelle Gunther, a traveler on this route long before me; Chris Jensen, Sybil and John Martin, Susan Miron, Susan Kahn, Hallie Cohen and Frank Levy, Leah Baigell and Henry Kon, Marilyn and Phil Wellons, Eva Harris and Kalman Glantz, Larry Harmon and Susannah Sirkin, Susan Mead, Paul Biss and Miriam Fried, Daniel Dayan and Rachel Rosenblum, Michael Rosenbluth and Ronnie Rosenberg, Bob Ramsay and Helga Stephenson.

Fourth, I thank my friends who not only nourished me, but read and corrected this book. They include artist Susan

Erony, whose cover matches the excellence of her *mandelbrot*; my writing partner Helen Fremont, who read many versions of these pages; Mary Bralove, Margo Jefferson, Eva Fogelman, Etha Frenkel, Nora Frenkiel, Patricia Hampl, Dr. Nadine Koff, Laurel Leff, Susan Hecker Ray, Susan Reverby, Rochelle Rubinstein and Connie Shuman. To Sarah Miniaci, special thanks.

Fifth, my indomitable former classmates from Hunter College High School, Class of 1965, especially emergency physician Dr. Audrey Konow, and attorney/ice skater Linnea Levine. Many of them shared their past and ongoing cancer experiences with me and their correspondence over two years was invaluable.

Last here but first in all other categories, my partner in life and love Patrick Mehr, who literally saved my life, and makes it happier every day.

Also by Helen Epstein

Children of the Holocaust: Conversations with Sons and Daughters of Survivors

Where She Came From: A Daughter's Search for her Mother's History

The Long Half-Lives of Love and Trauma

A Jewish Athlete: Swimming Against Stereotype in 20th Century Europe

Archivist on a Bicycle

Joe Papp: An American Life

Music Talks: The Lives of Classical Musicians

Under A Cruel Star: A Life in Prague, 1941-1968 by Heda Margolius Kovály (English translation)

Made in the USA
Middletown, DE
12 October 2022

12575316R00116